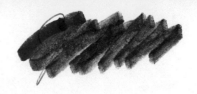

WHY I
SURVIVE
AIDS

Niro Markoff Asistent

with Paul Duffy

A FIRESIDE BOOK

Published by Simon & Schuster

New York   London   Toronto   Sydney
Tokyo   Singapore

F

Simon & Schuster/Fireside

Simon & Schuster Building
Rockefeller Center
1230 Avenue of the Americas
New York, New York 10020

Designed by Laurie Jewell
Manufactured in the United States of America

10   9   8   7   6   5   4   3   2   1   PBK

Library of Congress Cataloging in Publication Data
Asistent, Niro Markoff, date
Why I survive AIDS / Niro Markoff Asistent : with Paul Duffy.
p. cm.
Includes bibliographical references.
1. Asistent, Niro Markoff, date—Health.   2. AIDS (Disease)—
Patients—United States—Biography.   3. Healing.   I. Duffy, Paul.
II. Title.
RC607.A26A85   1991
362.1'9697'920092—dc20   91-20453
CIP
0-671-68352-7 (pbk)

The ideas, procedures and suggestions in this book are not
intended as a substitute for the medical advice of a trained
health professional. All matters regarding your health
require medical supervision. Consult your physician before
adopting the suggestions in this book, as well as about any
condition that may require diagnosis or medical attention.
The authors and publisher disclaim any liability arising
directly or indirectly from the use of this book.

Acknowledgments

TO ALL of my clients and workshop participants, thank you for your endless courage and willingness to discover a new way of living and dying. You are the wind beneath my wings.

To Barbara Gess, my insightful editor, thank you for presenting me with this amazing opportunity, which has been both a great challenge and a wonderful gift.

To Geraldine, thank you for being there when I needed you. To Manahar and Joan, thank you for your editorial assistance.

To my family, thank you, Ivan, Taty, Anny, and Nadine for your constant love and support. Thank you Papa for the endless rainbow of inspiration you brought to my life and to you Mom. The love and friendship we share today is concrete proof that miracles can happen.

To the men in my life, thank you, Vasant, Gawain, George, Doudou, Paul Lowe, Amitabh, and Jeru for being my teachers and friends. *Namasté.*

To the women in my life, thank you, Aurora, Delphine, Patricia, Mradula, and Masha for our shared conspiracy of laughter, tears, and celebration of the goddess energy.

To my precious children, Tanguy and Barbara. You are my true masters. Thank you for putting up with me and for your endless faith in me.

And finally to you, Paul. Without you this book would not have been possible. I am grateful that you are in my life. Thank you, my friend.

To Nado
to Osho
and . . . Amitabh

Contents

To say yes you have to sweat,
roll up your sleeves,
and plunge both hands into life
up to your elbows.
It is easy to say no,
even if saying no means death.

—JEAN ANOUILH,
Antigone

Foreword

IT IS TRULY an honor to be asked to write a few words of introduction for Niro Markoff Asistent's book, *Why I Survive AIDS*. Not only is it a remarkable book for patients with AIDS, but truly for any human being who is willing to look at themselves and grow; get rid of the old; and start a new life minus the old traumas, the outdated conditioning, and the leftover scars and pain—they are no longer necessary for survival.

This book really touched old buttons which I thought I had resolved and which I still need to work on! And although some of the techniques that come so easily to Niro, as an experienced meditator, may not be everybody's cup of tea, maybe it's time for us to try a new brand of tea!

Niro's story about her own discovery of the AIDS disease as well as her struggle with it—step-by-step—is a light in the darkness for millions. This is especially so because it is not a book of "how to heal," not a "recipe" for recovery, but a simply written account of a remarkable life filled with pain, hurt, frustration, hope, and the slow beginning of an awareness of how to change your life without miracle cures and "tools" from outside, but by becoming aware of all our *inner* resources and *inborn* gifts. What Niro has to say about forgiveness and the New Age trap is enormously helpful—we don't need to add guilt by implying that patients create their own diseases (cancer included). This is a great book, a beacon of light and a guide to millions of our PWAs, showing them again that AIDS does not have to be a fatal illness but can be a gateway to a new and healthier, happier life.

To Life!!!

ELISABETH KÜBLER-ROSS, M.D.

WHY I
SURVIVE
AIDS

1

MY JOURNEY

1

An Invitation

MY NAME is Niro. I am a woman who has lived through a powerful, and life-transforming experience. In November 1985, I tested positive for the human immune deficiency virus (HIV) and was diagnosed with AIDS-related complex (ARC). I had been infected by my lover, Nado, who was unaware that he was carrying the virus.

While I had been completely denying my condition, the symptoms of this disease of our time had already been ravaging my body for at least a year. In reaction to my diagnosis, I vacillated between deep numbness and extreme rage. Ultimately I surrendered, and accepted the unacceptable: death. In that instant, I recognized that I could no longer pretend that I was not personally accountable for my physical condition. I will always be grateful to my doctor for admitting that there was nothing he could do, because his honesty forced me to take responsibility for my own life.

I realized that I had a finite number of days left to live—approximately five hundred, if I was lucky. Each day was now very precious, so I rearranged my priorities, and put myself on the top of the list. Up until that point in my life, I had always denied my needs, playing the role of the caretaker to my parents, my husband, my children, and even my spiritual master. Having nothing left to lose, I decided to use my disease as a final opportunity for learning and growth, instead of being victimized by it. I embarked on a journey to discover who I am, not in relation to the world outside, but in terms of my true essence within. It was the beginning of the most important journey of my life.

By May 1986 I was symptomless, and in full remission from ARC. To my surprise, I even tested HIV antibody negative, and have remained so ever since. Nine months later, my lover Nado peacefully healed into death.

I feel as though I have lived a miracle, and I am still deeply grateful to the mystery of it. The true miracle of my healing is that I never tried to heal myself. Back in 1985, due to the hysteria of the media and the medical community, an AIDS-related diagnosis was virtually a death sentence. It is my belief that it is because I totally accepted that I would die, and began living in the moment, that I am still alive today.

Inspired by this experience, I created the Foundation for S.H.A.R.E. (the Self Healing AIDS-Related Experiment) to share my experience with others and to help change the limited belief that AIDS is one-hundred-percent fatal. I knew in my heart that if I could do it, others could as well, and I dedicated myself to making my "rare" experience commonplace. Fortunately, more and more people are realizing that AIDS is a chronic condition, and a major opportunity for personal and planetary transformation.

The first part of this book is the story of my own arduous journey of learning how to trust what I knew and what I did not know about healing. Along the way, I often fell backward into self-doubt and despair. At times I still fall, as you may during your journey. This journey has its ups and downs, left and right turns, great insights and deep doubts in the ceaseless motion of self-healing.

The second part of the book is based on my work as a facilitator, and is inspired by the humble and courageous individuals I have had the privilege of working with. It is not a magical formula, a set of ironclad rules, or a strict regimen for healing; rather it is a sharing of insights, lessons, and tools that can guide you to discover and trust your own healer within. The premise of the book is that you know better than anyone else the direction of your healing path.

For many of us faced with the challenge of a life-threatening condition, the reality of healing is very difficult and overwhelming. It is a journey of despair and hope, fear and trust, anger and vulnerability, including the rage we sometimes feel toward God and others for "abandoning" us. Yet the healing process, as many of you may have already discovered, cannot be forced. Along my journey I discovered a paradox:

Healing is an allowing, not a doing, yet we need to do everything we can physically, emotionally, and spiritually to help that allowing to happen.

Allowing is the willingness to let go and to suspend what we think is or isn't possible. Healing occurs when we let go of the past, accept the present, and open ourselves to the mystery of the future. Life then becomes an exciting adventure, a valued learning experience, and a source of great expansion. Yet, before we can truly experience this expansion, we need to say yes to our resistance and contraction. By accepting our contraction, by saying yes to our no, we simply accept what is so. By accepting the contraction, we move beyond duality to see the dance between contraction and expansion. There is no other way to move beyond it—first being aware of no, and then accepting it. For most of us this requires tremendous trust, shifting from our rational mind to our intuitive mind.

It was through my intuition that I realized the connection between the physical body and the emotions—a connection that many doctors are now discovering through the science of psychoimmunology. As I explored my emotional pain and fear, I discovered not only the source of imbalance that led to my dis-ease, but also what to do to support my healing. By tuning in to the source of the mind-body connection, we can offer our body the opportunity to respond. For some of us the response may be a healing on the physical level, and for others it may be a healing on the emotional level, preparing us for a completion into death.

My intuition also told me that this condition was my "wake-up call." I could have chosen either to respond to the message or to roll over and go back to sleep. I chose to wake up. Every crisis, whether it be illness, the consequences of addiction, or the loss of a loved one, offers us an opportunity to wake up. It is like an earthquake. It is life's way of shaking us up. What I mean is this: Life punched me in the face so forcefully that I was unable to escape the shocking reality. My reactions ranged from numbness to anger to despair and finally to soul-searching questioning.

As I questioned my life, I realized that I had spent the majority of it asleep. I had forgotten who I am and why I am here. I was moving through life unconsciously, like a sophisticated robot. My diagnosis served as a wonderful tool to assist me in examining the limitations of my conditioning.

I had never taken the time to question my early conditioning and the personality I had created based on it. It was time to examine these things honestly, keeping what still served me and discarding what was no longer appropriate. I began to take responsibility for my life from that new state of awareness, moving from the indulgence of the victim to the integrity of the master.

Many people, faced with a similar crisis, have not yet discovered the gift of accepting the wake-up call that their body is sending them. All they want is for the symptoms to go away. In fact, they are willing to endure the most extreme and expensive treatments to rid themselves of the condition.

This is because we are a society of people who will do anything to avoid being uncomfortable. We go to the doctor, who gives us painkiller to kill the pain, and to the psychiatrist, who gives us pills to alter our moods. We seek out the priest, who promises salvation, and the guru, who points to enlightenment. We're anesthetized during the miracle of childbirth, repress cold symptoms which are actually our body's way of cleansing itself, and keep ourselves busy with all kinds of re-creation to escape the loneliness and despair we feel inside. We do personal-growth workshops, read self-help books, and meditate to transcend the darkness and live in the light. We'll do anything to avoid the discomfort of our physical and emotional pain, even if it means denying who we are. In our society being uncomfortable is not considered "natural."

For example, try this exercise. Clasp your hands, webbing

your fingers together. Feel how natural and effortless it feels. Now separate your fingers, move them over one, and clasp your hands again. Now notice how it feels. Does it feel strange and uncomfortable? Do you find yourself wondering how long you will have to maintain this position, and when you will be able to cross your fingers in their "natural" position again? Often what we think of as natural is merely what we are used to, and what is comfortable. We confuse the natural with the familiar. Healing requires a willingness to let go of the "naturalness" of what is familiar and to say yes to the discomfort of what is new.

Since I began my own healing journey, I have worked as a facilitator with hundreds of people, and we all have one thing in common. Eventually we arrive at an aspect of our condition that is not comfortable. At that point there are two choices. One is to build a wall of resistance, denial, or postponement, to say no. The other is to finally say yes to the condition, with all of its pain and frightening feelings. As you read this book, I invite you to approach your healing from a new place, one that may not be familiar, but that may be far more natural than you realize.

This is the essence of healing. To learn to say yes to what is, instead of trying to change it to how we would like it to be. I invite you to question what your condition is about, and to discover what it can teach you, before you try to get rid of it. Often, when we receive the lesson our illness or condition is teaching us, the teacher can go away.

This book is an invitation to go beyond what feels good, what feels comfortable, and at the same time to be gentle with yourself. Create an environment in which you feel nourished and safe. Give yourself permission to participate fully in the processes in the second half of the book. They are designed to provide you with a new approach toward yourself, your life, and your dis-ease, and have succeeded in doing that for hundreds of people who have participated in my workshops.

I invite you to welcome your condition as your wake-up call, the perfect tool to assist you in reaching your maximum potential.

Perhaps one day, if you aren't already, you may find yourself grateful to your condition for creating this opportunity in your life. I invite you to say yes to your condition. To say yes to who you are. To say the healing yes.

In love and light we heal,

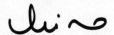

2

Prelude
to My Path

THE INTRICATE and winding road that led to my healing journey was uniquely mine, just as your path is unique to you. My journey began in Belgium in 1945, where I was born Yvette Markoff to Pierre Markoff, a handsome White Russian of aristocratic background, and Christianne de Rode, a beautiful upper-middle-class Belgian woman. Growing up, I was aware of the difference between my conservative mother and her family, and my intense, seeking father. (He had been forced to flee Russia during the revolution, and never saw his family again.) I had never identified with the Belgian name Yvette, and so when I was thirteen, I changed it to Masha, a name I felt more accurately reflected my own intense Russian nature.

My mother dedicated her life to her brilliant, demanding husband, whom she did not understand very well. Her dream was to give birth to the son he longed for, and both my parents hoped I would be a boy. But I was the third of three daughters. This unrealized expectation set the tone for what would become a major theme of my life: rejection. In terms of my parents' wishes, I was simply the wrong gender. (As an adult, I was the wrong gender to my male bisexual lover as well.) I grew up with a sense of not being accepted for who I was. I often had difficulty standing up for myself, and saying no to the demands of others, even when it went against my own sense of integrity.

The world I remember as a child was that of a suppressed matriarchy in which all the women—my mother, my grandmother, my aunt, and my sisters—devoted their lives to satisfying the needs of their men. Service to the family, and to the men who provided for it, was so ingrained in us, that I had no concept that there could be another way. In fact, today I still carry a deep respect for that attitude. I sincerely believe that if more of us lived in service, for a universal purpose and not just for personal gain, the planet would be a warmer place.

I have always been a spiritual seeker. As a child I was very mystical, and quickly became alienated from the conventional adults around me. As a teenager, while studying Catholic catechism, I began having psychic experiences. I understood theology from a different perspective than that of the superficial interpretations imposed on me by my teachers. I considered my relationship to God as personal, and I experienced my own individual connection to what I knew as the Source of Infinite Love.

I discovered very early on that I could use disease as a tool to manipulate those around me. If I was unhappy, or didn't want to go to school, I would terrify my parents by paralyzing my legs, or creating some other childhood illness. It was the perfect way to escape, and it still is.

Whenever I was ill, my mother pampered me by making me lemonade, allowing me to read my favorite books, and sharing time alone with me. When I saw that I received my mother's affection basically only when I was ill, I recognized the power of disease. In fact, everyone in my family seemed to pay more attention to me when I was ill, so I played the role of the sick child for years.

My use of disease as a manipulative tool was not something I originated on my own. Both my mother and father were sick during a majority of my childhood. My father was diagnosed manic-depressive, and received chemical treatment through the majority of his life. My mother suffered from rheumatic fever, and spent eleven months in bed when I was nine years old. Disease became a major tool of survival for me because somewhere deep down I surmised that I had to compete for my parents' attention. If they stopped caring for me because they were too ill, or because I wasn't "good enough" (i.e., because I was the wrong gender), or for whatever reason, I would literally die. I'm not suggesting my parents had any intention of abandoning me, but this childhood fear of abandonment is still with me today.

While growing up in Belgium shortly after the Second World War, I was raised to conform to the social etiquette of our culture. By the time I was a teenager I had become a very elegant robot. Since childhood I have wanted to "be in service to the world." I studied social science with the intention of working with children in Third World countries, but my family prohibited me from doing that. Instead I worked with abused children in my own homeland and as a volunteer in the Service Civile Internationale, Europe's equivalent to the Peace Corps.

I escaped from the prison of my home life into an unexpected pregnancy and marriage with Nicholas Steinbach, a young jet-setter who was as violent as he was charming. Although I do not regret marrying him, I see now that it was a doomed decision for both of us. We were too young to take on the responsibility of being parents or to understand the true commitment of marriage. Our fragile love was not able to withstand the constant pressure we both felt because of our own sense of frustration and insecurity. Nicholas was afraid of not being able to be a proper provider for his budding family, and imprisoned himself within that role. I was a prisoner of the way things "should be," and was living in a constant state of frustration. Even though I loved him at the time, our relationship was not a healthy one. We would explode in anger at each other for the most trivial reasons. It was a perfect illustration of how a relationship can die because two people are unable truly to communicate with each other. The only good that came out of it was my two beautiful children. Four unbearable years of marriage with Nicholas left me physically and emotionally abused. I finally left him, fearing for my sanity and for the well-being of my children. I know now that, had I stayed, I would long since be dead, either by his hand or my own.

As a single mother I was tremendously overstressed, trying to perform as father, mother, provider, and homemaker at the same time. Even though I "wore the pants" in the family, the little girl inside of me longed to find a man whom I could serve and who would take care of me. Not being able to find such a man, I shut down.

I forgot what I genuinely wanted from life, besides providing the best for my children and following the basic principles of a "normal" life. A part of me was so insecure that I fell into the trap of the "designer" lifestyle, donning the mask of a jet-setter in order to find my self-esteem. The little girl inside of me believed that if I did all the glamorous and exciting things that the magazines and T.V. shows promoted, then it was a sign of my personal "success."

I began a lifestyle based on exploring my connection with men, and enjoyed the novelty of letting myself be taken care of by my admirers. I was not yet aware of the cost of the game of manipulating my physical beauty to get my material needs met. At the time it all looked good from the outside. I was in with the right people at the right time, in the right places, wearing the right clothes—and yet, underneath, I was suffocating from the superficiality of it all. In that world, material success was religion, and money was respected like the golden calf. It felt as if I were withering away from the tremendous lack of spiritual love. Because I was doubting my jet-setter lifestyle, I felt even more insecure, believing that something must be wrong with me. Instead of trusting what I knew deep in my heart (that life was pushing me to search within for the answers), I denied my natural flow and became a boring people-pleaser.

Eventually, my inner emptiness became too much for me. I gave up my "designer life" and, like so many generations of Europeans before me, emigrated to America. I moved to New York City and took a job as a manager in a health-food restaurant owned by a friend. He introduced me to est training, which had a great impact on my life because it taught me to access a new level of integrity within. I quickly became a guest seminar leader, and volunteered for the organization, although it didn't really fill the spiritual void I was feeling.

Another friend had told me about his spiritual master, but for months I paid him no mind. One night he invited me to a video screening of this self-realized, enlightened master. I was curious, and decided to go. I'll never forget the first time I saw Osho, a small Indian man with intensely powerful eyes. My heart cracked open, and I immediately knew I would become his disciple. I would follow his teachings and guidance, using him as an anchor to take the journey of self-discovery. Several months later, I traveled to his main ashram (a community where people live and practice the teachings of a spiritual master) on the West Coast to be in his "Buddha field of energy." The day I arrived, he drove by in his car. As he passed, he looked into my eyes, into my soul, and that spiritual void I had felt all my life was filled. I felt like I had finally come "home." I became his disciple, or sannyasin, as he called it, the following day, and was given the name Anand Niro, an Indian Sanskrit name which means "bliss water."

While at Osho's ashram I received my training as a facilitator in gestalt, primal, and breath therapy, as well as in various meditation techniques and energy balancing. The active meditations that Osho designed for the modern Western man not only allowed me to release years of blocked emotional energy repressed within my physical body, but opened my heart as well. I still use many of Osho's meditations in the workshops I lead, and as I will share later, his presence in my life played a major role in my healing journey.

Because I traveled to the main ashram only a few times a year, I stayed connected to its energy by creating my own meditation center in my apartment. Several of my fellow sannyasins would join me for evening meditations and satsangs (a gathering in which we would listen to the words of the master, then sing and dance in celebration). Some sannyasins were traveling to or from the main ashram, and would spend the night. Others would stay over for several days, sometimes weeks, to "be in the energy." My apartment became too small, so we rented a house just outside of the city. There was room for twenty-five residents, but it soon grew to sixty. We finally moved to a magnificent castle in New Jersey, and our meditation center was born.

I was living one of my childhood dreams. I was a successful director of one of the largest meditation centers on the East Coast.

I was living with other spiritual seekers like myself, many of whom I dearly loved. I was living a "life in service," working as a spiritual therapist, and I was raising my two children in an atmosphere of open love.

Because the circumstances of my life fit the pictures of the vision I held as a child, it was difficult for me to acknowledge that part of me that still was not fulfilled. Even though I was meditating every day, had surrendered to my beloved master, and had renounced the superficial materialistic world, I was still feeling those "negative emotions" such as loneliness and despair.

I would use a tremendous amount of energy trying to hide or get rid of my dark feelings. I would meditate even more, to reach that sense of inner bliss, or use the various therapy techniques available to me to escape the pain. Even though I had achieved my dream, it did not bring me what my soul was longing for: namely, to find my soul partner and merge.

Then I met Nado.

Nado and I had a relationship that can only be described as destiny. The first time I laid eyes on him was at a sannyasin party. His energy was intense, and although I was curious about him, I chose not to speak to him. A few days later I was invited to a meditation evening in Brooklyn. As I entered the loft and was greeted by the host, I was pleasantly surprised to discover that it was Nado. The connection between us was obvious, yet we realized it arose from a deep sense of recognition, rather than a romantic attraction.

After the meditation, Nado rushed up to me and rudely asked me why I had changed my hairstyle to its present short length and dark color. At first I thought he was someone I had known when I was younger and my hair was long and blond, but he quickly explained that, although we had never met (in this life at least), between the ages of five and seventeen, he had had a recurring dream about me in which I had long blond hair. Seeing me materialized in the flesh in his loft that evening quite frankly blew his mind.

During our first days together, we discovered we had a lot in common. Because he was Dutch, not only did we share our European upbringing but also the feeling of being separated from our history and homeland by the great Atlantic Ocean. He had also studied the social and political sciences in college, and our taste in art was practically identical. We shared a passion for the surrealist painter Magritte, the choreographer Béjart, and the genius composer Bach. Our most important connection was that we were both seekers of truth and shared a deep love for our master Osho.

Our attraction to each other was not love at first sight in the usual romantic sense. Nado was married to a friend of mine, and even though they were separated at the time, I never considered him as a potential partner. One day another friend at the center casually observed that our budding relationship seemed more than platonic. She referred to the way in which Nado would hover around me, serving me tea and bringing me flowers. I suppose I was blind to the signals at the time, since I was so busy taking care of a myriad of details at the center.

My birthday arrived and I considered having a party. I asked myself who I wanted to invite and to my surprise I realized that the only person I wanted to share my birthday with was Nado. He arrived that evening cradling a spray of white orchids. We gazed knowingly at each other, gently kissed, and then giggled innocently like two children on a first date. Under a full moon in July, we spent what became the first of many nights together. The next morning, before Nado left for work, I invited him to move in with me. The fact that he was still legally married, and that there were rumors that he might be gay, had no influence over the simple loving feelings I had for him.

When I suggested that moving in together could be our first step to growing old together, he quickly retorted, "Don't count on me, I won't be around." Of course my feelings were immediately hurt, because I assumed he meant he was planning on eventually leaving me. Sensing my contraction, he explained that he would not be around to see old age because he would be dead by the age of forty-two. I was startled by the seriousness of his tone, and inquired further. He shared with me that he had intuitively known since he was a boy that he would die in his forty-second year.

At first Nado was very sexual with me, in a tender and passionate way, dispelling any question in my naïve mind that he was anything but one-hundred-percent heterosexual. After several months, however, the honeymoon waned and Nado withdrew his physical affection from me. In an effort to avoid feeling rejected, I rationalized his sudden distance from me as his need for creative space (he was a brilliant poet and dancer). Yet deep down I knew it was more than that. He began to avoid me in other areas as well. Every time I addressed the subject of sex and our growing separation from each other he would leave the room.

After several months together, we began practicing "safe sex," because it was advocated by our master at the ashram. Osho was a pioneer in terms of the safe sex guidelines. By 1984, everyone at the ashram was required to practice safe sex. We used not only condoms, but rubber gloves as well. The running joke between sannyasins was, "How's your glove life?" French kissing was also not allowed. Can you imagine how difficult and frustrating it was, after having normal relations with your lover, not to be able to French-kiss anymore? It took complete unconditional trust in our master, and a lot of will power.

I personally believe that, because of Nado's own fear of rejection, he closed the door to our brief and fragile connection and hid behind it as a way of protecting his secret. I quickly realized that his conflict about his sexual identity, and his fear of intimacy, were taboo subjects. Instead of talking about it in a healthy, open way, I internalized our struggle, and hid the constant pain I felt as a result of the resistance and separation that was now between us.

In the hope of saving our relationship, I repressed my feelings and tolerated Nado's rejection of me even though he avoided any intimate sexual contact with me for weeks at a time. Because our connection was so strong, and my commitment to that connection so total, leaving Nado was not an option. I had made a vow to myself that, since Nado and I were soul mates, we were destined to live our lives together till death should part us, regardless of how much I was starving emotionally and sexually.

Interestingly enough, I was also starving myself physically. Although at the time I was a "strict" vegetarian, my diet consisted almost exclusively of French bread, cappuccino, and Belgian chocolate, with lots of Häagen-Dazs ice cream for dessert. (I was a connoisseur of international vegetarian cuisine!) Although there were deliciously nutritious vegetarian meals available at the center, I chose to starve my body by feeding my indulgence.

My weakness for Belgian chocolate, an addiction which I am still battling today, stems back to my childhood, when I received a daily ration of chocolate from my Dad as a sign of approval. Not only was such poor nutrition a reaction to my undernourished and overstressed life (I was looking for emotional nourishment), but it actually contributed to the depression I was feeling. I ended up gaining twenty-five pounds in less than a month as a reaction to Nado losing his attraction to me. At least if I was fat, he would have a valid reason.

I realize now how cruel I was being to myself. Much like the women in my family who suppressed their uniqueness in deference to their men, I was denying who I was, in service to a romantic idea of relationship. I grew from being a vibrant, expressive, and extroverted woman into a repressed, withdrawn, and shameful little girl convinced that I was no longer desirable. I beat myself up for failing to create a safe space for Nado to express his internal struggle, and I felt guilty for losing our connection. It felt like my cherished dream of Nado and me sharing our lives as soul partners had escaped beyond my reach. It was as if it were tottering precariously on a shelf far above me, and the circumstances of my life were rocking me in such a way that the dream was destined to fall and shatter into a million pieces.

3

Strange Symptoms, Shattered Dreams

IN MAY 1984, my body responded to the stress and emotional drain in my life by becoming extremely sick. I knew something very important was happening to me, but I didn't know what. The symptoms were strange and puzzling. Every afternoon around four o'clock my body tensed and began shaking. My breathing constricted and my temperature rose to 104°. For weeks I vacillated between high fevers and clammy chills, waking up every night in perspiration-soaked bedclothes.

One of the most agonizing symptoms was a throbbing pain in my neck, arms, and legs. At times it was so intense that my entire body would contract. I would hold my breath and wait for the pain to pass, for what seemed like hours. Fortunately I remembered from my training as a facilitator that if I held my breath I would hold in the pain as well, so I forced myself to close my eyes and breathe deeply. As I inhaled and exhaled consciously, my body would shake intensely as it allowed the release of the physical pain. There were times when the pain would attack while I was driving, and I had to pull over to the side of the road and let my body shake.

I became more and more exhausted as the symptoms increased. The fevers would literally knock me out. The staff doctor at the meditation center was unable to diagnose my strange symptoms, and sent me for some tests. The only condition that could be determined was a severe urinary infection, for which I was prescribed antibiotics. For months, the symptoms persisted. After a while I became accustomed to the feverish chills and the semicomatose states I would fall into every night.

I had very little energy left during the day to fulfill my duties as the center coordinator. Ironically, I had created the center so that I could live in peace and harmony with other sannyasins like myself. Yet, because I wanted to please my master, I was obsessed with doing everything perfectly. My daily schedule was backbreaking. On a typical day I would wake up at six A.M., supervise the morning meditation, and then work nonstop as a therapist, administrator, bookkeeper, and staff supervisor until midnight, when I would fall into bed exhausted. No wonder I assumed that the extreme exhaustion I felt for months was simply my body's reaction to my intense schedule. Because I wanted to do everything perfectly, I often pushed myself too far.

When I became sick, I also approached my condition with a very tough attitude, pushing myself even farther, and ignoring the intense signals that my body was sending me. I kept pretending that it was nothing, which was my way of dealing with my fear. I only knew how to push more and be more demanding of myself and of those around me. A cacophony of extremely critical voices in my head—voices that sounded like my parents, my teachers, and my ex-husband—kept telling me: "You are not good enough. You should be doing more, faster, and better." I was a prisoner of all the "should"s in my life. That panel of judgmental voices was a constant source of stress, and robbed me of any joy I might have experienced.

The fact that the doctors could not find a specific cause for my symptoms or make a concrete diagnosis steered me away from searching for a medical solution. I figured that, since I was living in a meditation center, I would search inside myself, embark on an inner quest, to discover what was happening to me.

Today, I realize that it was more of a trial than a quest, and that I was the unforgiving and uncompassionate judge. Within my own mind, I tried and sentenced myself with a litany of accusations that showed why I deserved to be sick. I didn't eat right, I didn't meditate enough, I wasn't exercising enough. I wasn't doing enough of this or enough of that; if only I was doing more of this or that . . .

This barrage of "should"s and "should not"s was constantly

making me feel like a failure, and I would resent my painful body even more. I could not find compassion or acceptance toward what was happening in me. My old habit of self-judgment was slowly and meticulously destroying me.

I also rationalized my condition from a metaphysical perspective. At the time I believed that the symptoms were a manifestation of the breaking of my ego, a goal which I had been determined to accomplish. It was another one of the many "should"s I had taken upon myself when I became a disciple. As a disciple of Osho, we are encouraged to be in the world but not of it. Rather than living a monastic lifestyle, we actively participated in the marketplace, but did so in a constant state of meditation.

I was still caught up in the process of validating myself through what I was doing rather than through who I was being. Because I was determined to please others, especially my master, I would do anything to serve that end. I allowed myself very little time to just be and enjoy life. I now understand what Osho meant when he invited us to "stop swimming up the river of life and go with the flow," but at the time it was very important for me to stay in control. In fact, I was so stuck in the "control mode," trying desperately to direct all the events in my life, that I used to actually "push the river." The less I felt in control of my relationship with Nado, the more I would exert control over the other circumstances of my life. I wanted to be so "good" that I continued to deny the message my body was sending me even as the illness progressed.

I was very scared, yet unable to reach out for any kind of help. Whenever my friends or colleagues inquired about my physical and emotional health, I courageously answered that I was fine, never really sharing how lost and powerless I felt. I was ashamed of being sick, and believed that, as the center coordinator, I had to present a certain image of having it all together. I perceived my illness as a weakness, believing that I would be betraying the center by not being available to work twenty-four hours a day nonstop.

Because of this self-imposed image, I felt extremely isolated. I didn't trust what I was feeling, and didn't feel safe enough with anyone else to share what was happening. I did not know how to say simply that I was terrified that the pain in my legs and my arms, and the strange trembling fits, might be a sign of a serious illness. The only person I felt I could be open with was Nado, yet it was too disturbing for him to see me sick. Like many partners of people suffering from illness, he felt helpless. Rather than make my beloved uncomfortable, I chose to keep my fears to myself. I protected Nado, my kids, and my friends from the truth. I wore the mask of "everything is fine" as a way to take care of them. Deep down, I secretly wished I could let down my mask and finally let myself be taken care of, but I was afraid of falling apart. There I was in the same old place, trapped by a warped sense of responsibility, with no way out. I needed a break badly. I needed to escape the dream I had created, which had descended into a nightmare.

The sicker I became, the more I wanted to feel close to Nado, and to feel protected by him. I needed so much to be reassured in some way, but the more I wanted it, the more it seemed to push him away. I had an enormous need to be held by Nado. Instead of simply expressing it to him, I constantly analyzed myself out of it, judging it as a need I didn't have a right to feel. As a result, I often tried to covertly manipulate him into holding me. If he refused, I would feel that I wanted to get even with him, but I usually ended up feeling horrible as well.

Our relationship became more and more strained, and we grew distant from each other. We were no longer speaking the same language, and it hurt so much. Because it was Nado's affection I craved, I was not interested in relating to the others at the center. My interaction with them became artificial and forced. Ironically, I closed the door to my family and friends when I needed support the most.

You might honestly question why I stayed for so long in such a self-destructive relationship. It was never my intention to reach that stage. I did not decide, "Okay, this time let's have a real destructive, harmful relationship." Both Nado and I tried very hard, yet we kept missing each other. I suppose it had a lot to do with the conditioning of our childhoods.

For Nado, it was his belief that his bisexuality was "wrong." Eventually I became a mirror for his own self-judgment. The more he shrouded his "other life" in secrecy, becoming defensive upon inquiry, the more contracted I would become. This contraction or withdrawal was my defensive reflex against the feeling of being betrayed. I never really judged his bisexuality, although I perceived it as a threat and a source of rejection. I also felt hurt that it created separation between us since he was not able to communicate with me about it.

For me, the idea of leaving Nado and ending up alone seemed more painful than enduring the relationship as it was. My tendency was to judge myself for not loving him right. Somehow I deluded myself into believing that if I behaved differently perhaps he would not need to seek affection from anyone else. If only I had been somebody else (a man, perhaps, like the son my father had wanted so badly), I would have been able to satisfy his sexual tendencies.

It was my old habit of seeing myself as wrong. I was unable to recognize my own needs, and stand up for them. By accepting this situation, I was literally abusing myself over and over. Having been verbally and emotionally and sometimes physically abused as a child, my only way to deal with such abuse was to pretend that it wasn't happening. This form of denial was imprinted deeply in me as my way to survive in the adult world, and fed the energy of the victim in me. I would seek the approval of others, continually excusing myself for just being alive. With this attitude, it was not surprising that I generated an abusive relationship in my marriage and later with Nado. Naïvely, I did not believe that it could be otherwise, even though secretly I clung to the dream that someday my savior would come, as all the romance novels and Hollywood movies had promised.

At times, fortunately, I found temporary comfort in meditation, because it grounded me. During meditation, the unbearable pain in my heart, which almost seemed to be the direct source of my physical pain, was bearable. There were even rare moments when it would actually disappear.

By July of 1984, two months after the strange symptoms began, we received orders from the head organization of the main ashram to close our center. Osho had decided that all of the centers in the United States would close, and only the main ashram would remain open. This news was very difficult for me to accept. I felt a deep sense of discouragement and failure. All the long hours and hard work I had spent realizing my dream now seemed like wasted energy.

After closing the center I decided to return to Europe with my children to complete some unfinished business there. I was anxious, tense, and unhappy all of the time, and I tried desperately to make those feelings disappear. My main tool was pretending. If I said enough times that everything was all right, maybe it would be. Then I would think that maybe everything actually was all right, and that I was a spoiled brat to want things to be different. I felt trapped in a vicious circle of mind games, and I began doubting my own sanity.

Throughout that period, everything I did required extra effort. As usual, I pushed myself beyond my limits, which were either nonexistent or ill-defined in the first place. I would impose challenges on myself, such as driving from Spain to Belgium in one stretch, because "I did not have enough money to stop in a hotel." I had a hundred crazy excuses that kept negating a simple human way to take care of myself. The more I said no to myself, the more resentment I had toward myself.

By winter I grew more and more dissatisfied with my life, and subsequently more and more sick. A local doctor diagnosed me with walking pneumonia. This period of my life was extremely difficult, and I was depressed most of the time. I was barely able to drag myself around, struggling for the sake of my children to keep up the pretense that everything was okay.

I didn't respect my own body enough to listen to the constant signals it was sending me. I never took the time simply to sit and ask myself: "What is really happening, right now? What am I feeling?" and put that information into perspective. I always pushed it away because I did not want to upset my children or the others in my family, or because I had to take care of business. I was living my life according to some arbitrary standard that "it was never the right time," according to the dictates of "circumstances" or "partner" or "country." I can see today what a powerful defense system it was. It was like putting a polish on everything to cover the dust; staying in the superficiality of the circumstances, simply because it felt safer.

Finally, during a breath therapy session with a colleague in Spain, I dropped the pretense that everything was okay. In breath therapy, you inhale and exhale continuously, creating a circle of breath, which builds up energy in the body and facilitates healing. While doing this, I began to release the streams of repressed emotion. I expressed the anger I felt toward myself for all the years of self-denial, and at Nado for not responding to our love. This was followed by a deep sadness, that we had missed the opportunity to merge, and truly love one another unconditionally. This was the first breakdown, when I began to face what was really happening.

After allowing the waves of emotion to be released, I felt empty, and open. In the silence of this emptiness I asked myself what was really happening with me. I was not so interested in easy answers, but in the question itself. I let myself be in the question. What was my body trying to tell me? How was I sabotaging myself? Who was it in me that was doing the sabotaging, and who was it in me asking the question? I felt fragile and vulnerable. I had begun to lift the veil of denial, open my eyes, and honestly view my life. I had taken the first step on my path of healing.

I returned to the States and moved to East Hampton, New York. Shortly thereafter, Nado came to visit and moved in again. Our reunion after months of separation was like a honeymoon. Unfortunately, he could not sustain his physical affection toward me, and it wore thin quickly. I fell backward into the illusion that I could control the circumstances and push the river of our love.

My old ways quickly overshadowed my new fragile openness and vulnerability. I no longer felt the magic of living in the question. The freedom of "I don't know" became imprisoned by the need to know and have it my way. My insecurity returned, burying that delicate sense of newness.

I can see now how my insecurity took control again, as a protection device. It created the illusion that I had authentic power over my life, when in reality my emotional life had become completely unmanageable. Although that attitude did serve as a filter to shield me from the shame and loneliness I felt inside, it was a very subtle way of sabotaging my intuition. My main response to life was, "No, I've had enough" or "How can I escape this?" At the time I was not conscious of my negative attitude, and it colored everything in my life. Every step seemed like a struggle, and required energy that did not seem to be available to me. The rare moments of harmony and joy I experienced came while I was meditating on the beach in the morning before work. Because of this I wanted to spend more time in meditation, and so I took a temporary sabbatical from my therapy practice.

That summer, Nado and I were hired as caretakers on a magnificent estate located right on the beach. The owner was only there on weekends, so our schedules were flexible during the week. It was a blessing. I needed time to think and to discover what I wanted to do with my life. I needed to reconcile myself with the change from communal living to living with my children as a nuclear family again. Because I was no longer running the meditation center, and I was living on the beach, life was much lighter and easier. As a result, my body felt much better, even though I still had very little energy and it was difficult to work. We lived a very simple life, Nado, my children, and I. In a way it was like beginning a new chapter.

But in September 1985 everything was thrown out the window with the results of Nado's HIV test. He had been routinely tested at the main ashram as part of a new screening program. The hierarchy of the ashram was concerned about the spread of AIDS amongst the disciples, and had decided to close the doors of the ashram to anyone who tested positive for HIV. Nado was tested with hundreds of others for verification of his assumed health. Unlike my own, his body showed no symptoms whatsoever. His test came back highly positive, and at that moment, suddenly, all my strange symptoms made frightening sense.

4

Why Me?

UP UNTIL this point in my life, AIDS had been a fiction. Even though we were well informed about AIDS and safe sex at the ashram, it was something that was happening to people "out there." At the time I didn't know very many gay people or I.V. drug users, so I never conceived of the possibility that it would enter my life.

In a panic, I went to see a doctor who was recommended by a sannyasin friend. I wanted someone very caring, and my friend assured me that this doctor was the right one for me since he practiced meditation and had traveled to India several times. I trusted him right away, and at our first meeting he recommended that I get tested at the Suffolk County Health Department, where I could be tested anonymously. At the time, there was a very real fear of losing employment or insurance due to an HIV-positive test result.

In 1985, being tested at a health-department clinic in New York meant waiting six weeks for the results, and those six weeks were hell. The fear was so intense that I could only deal with it through denial and occasional rage. I would not even entertain the notion that I could possibly have AIDS. Even though the symptoms I had been suffering from for months, including diarrhea, thrush, and night sweats, were considered major warning signs, I refused to draw the terrible conclusion. I would convince myself, over and over, that it was not so. During the rare moments when I would consider the possibility, I felt intense anger toward Nado for exposing me to a deadly virus, and for his inability to trust me enough to be open and honest with me.

When the day for the test results came, Nado and I arrived at the clinic early. While we waited in the car for our appointment, I passed the time by enjoying the serenity of the pastoral surroundings. I remember that it was an exquisitely beautiful day. A few minutes before our appointment, it dawned on me. "Stop fooling yourself," I thought. "You know the test results are positive. When you come out of the building your life will be totally different." I looked at the sky and the birds and all of the beautiful nature around me and I thought to myself, "Take a good look, Niro, because when you come out again nothing will look the same."

When Nado and I entered the room, I could hardly breathe. Our counselor was so sweet in trying to break the news as gently as possible. I could feel her personal regret at having to be the one to announce to us that we were both HIV-positive, as she handed us our test results as proof that the shocking news was true. (Three months later the results of the Red Cross blood tests Nado and I had taken earlier came by registered mail. They were also HIV-positive.)

The counselor then proceeded to explain that the test results did not mean that we would have to change our lifestyle right away, but that it would be appropriate to be monitored by a doctor. She gave us a booklet from the health department containing instructions on what steps could be taken to postpone death, but I chose not to read it. To tell you the truth, I didn't want to hear about it. All of the media were completely negative and destructive, denying any possibility of hope in their unequivocal statements that AIDS was fatal, and that there was no cure.

When she asked if we had any questions, I just wanted to run out of the building. Her tone was very compassionate, but that produced the opposite of the intended effect on me. I hated being treated as someone fragile. I wanted to run away, and be alone. I needed to let the news in, to integrate it. I was at a loss as to how to react. I wanted to scream, to cry, to get out of there. Instead I repressed my feelings and refused to cry. With a shallow voice I answered no. Nado asked how long we had to live, and she softly answered: approximately eighteen months, if we were lucky. She invited us to call her if we needed support, assuring us that she was there to help.

The news of the positive results of my HIV test did not really register. It was like some tragic soap opera. I had ARC, which stood for AIDS-related complex. What the hell did that mean? Guaranteed death . . . eighteen months to live if I was lucky. But worse than that, it meant being cast out of my spiritual community, ostracized by the people I loved most. My dream of eventually retiring and living at the ashram was impossible as long as I tested HIV-positive. I also feared being judged by others, and becoming a source of repulsion, a leper. That would be too much to face; I was afraid of rejection more than I was of death itself. It was all just too unbearable, and I fell into a state of numbness.

The following day I returned to my doctor with the results of my test. I arrived very tense and full of questions, trying to hide the intensity of my fears. The gentleness and care I felt from him immediately alleviated my anxiety. On that day he provided me with one of the major elements for my healing journey. I very candidly asked him if there was anything that could be done about my situation. I wanted desperately to get rid of this horrifying condition so that I could go "home" to the ashram. He responded honestly by saying, "I'm sorry, there's nothing I can do for you except be here whenever you need me. I know very little about AIDS, and unfortunately the medical profession has yet to discover a cure." He then gave me the name of a top specialist on Long Island for further consultation.

I was empowered by his honesty, and felt completely taken care of, because there was such good communication between us. There was no need for pretense or false solutions. I knew that he really cared, and that the truth about my condition would always be given to me. That was priceless to me. I felt seen, respected, and understood. I felt treated as an equal human being—a feeling I rarely experienced in the presence of doctors. Most of the time I felt more like an object of science being studied.

His honesty and integrity was like a seed which slowly sprouted and eventually blossomed in me. The honest readiness to accept the facts as they were presented to me, and the courage to stand up for my truth despite the circumstances, became key components of my healing. I thanked him for his frankness and support, informing him that I needed to reconcile the situation in my mind and examine what my options were before I made any decisions. I promised him that I would come see him whenever I felt I needed the anchor of his guidance.

After I returned home, the reality of the news set in. There was nothing I or anyone else could do. My first reaction was "No!"—refusing to believe it—followed by "Why me?" Virtually every HIV client I have worked with in therapy has shared the same response. It is so instinctive it is nearly a reflex. It is the natural reaction of the survivor in us. Denial of the news or of the condition itself, followed by anger and resistance to accepting responsibility for it in our lives. In the beginning, denial and resistance are healthy reactions, but we can quickly fall into the role of victim if we stay stuck in them.

There were two main reasons I remained stuck in the "Why me?" attitude. First, it was my tendency to compare my present situation with the past. I constantly obsessed about what I had "lost." Yet in truth, when I was healthy, like many of us, I took life for granted. It wasn't until I was faced with my imminent death that I began to appreciate the fragile gift of life. Second, I would imagine all the terrible things that would happen to my two children. Since they had grown up without a father, it was unbearable to imagine them being raised by "normal" people who did not have the same spirituality and level of consciousness that they did. This only added to the guilt I felt about contracting the disease in the first place. I began organizing my legal affairs, and prepared to draw up a will. I purchased the best life insurance I could, so that my children would be financially taken care of after my death.

In my mind I played over and over again the tragic scenario of a long, painful suffering, in which I was completely helpless, dying in some strange hospital bed. This, more than death itself, terrified me. Now not only did I have to deal with the physical symptoms of high fevers, chronic diarrhea, and excruciating pain, but I had to live with my past regrets and future fears as well. The emotional stress that resulted from these anxieties not only prohibited healing but, I believe, actually contributed to the symptoms of the disease itself. I felt that I had failed and that I was running out of time.

My response to my fears was to become utterly frantic. I ran around like the proverbial chicken with her head cut off. Because I felt so helpless, I attempted to fix everything else around me. I compulsively cleaned the house from top to bottom. I became overprotective of my children, now in their teens, giving them unwanted advice and driving them crazy. I tried to communicate with Nado, to get him to talk, to get him to change—anything to avoid facing the terror I felt inside. My only way to survive the fear was to say no to my nightmare, and to the illness that was the source of it. At one point I called the specialist whom my doctor had recommended. After I explained my symptoms to his receptionist, she replied that I was not sick enough, and I would have to wait two months for an appointment.

For at least three weeks following the diagnosis, I vacillated between total numbness and intense anger. There were times when I was lost in a fog and nothing made sense. Then there were times when it would lift and I would experience intense rage at everything around me. The anger would come in waves, followed by accusation and blame, which would rise with it like the tide. I would usually blame Nado or use the old excuse that my body was betraying me. I blamed my body for getting sick, for not being strong enough, for leading me into temptation. Anything to avoid taking responsibility myself. An example of this was a letter I wrote to my body on one of my more difficult days.

An Open Letter To My Body

Today, you are really taking me for a total trip. You hurt everywhere, and my feet and fingers are so swollen I can hardly put on my Birkenstocks, and there's no way that I can put on my rings. I fucking ache everywhere, and then like a total dodo, I step on the scale, and I am ten pounds heavier. My morale drops below basement level. This is not at all funny. Here I am barely eating any sugar and this is the reward I get! Fuck you!

You have become my enemy. (The truth is you have been my enemy for a long time.) I remember when you grew too big too quickly, and I was told I was too tall to be a dancer. Then you blossomed and became very beautiful, creating so many problems for me. I didn't know how to handle all those men, and I had nobody to talk to. I felt the constant judgments of the women in my family, like I did something wrong, but I knew not what.

My relationship with you was one of ignorance. (I did not even have a full orgasm or discover masturbation until I was much older, that's how cut off we were from each other.) I could only use you through disease. The only time you ever gave me any satisfaction was when you were sick, and I would finally receive some attention. Oh, of course when I was eating too.

My affair with food started when I left home to live with my grandmother. At home, I used to hate eating what my mother served and I was slender. The only thing I liked was chocolate, and it was rarely available. Whenever we received it as an acknowledgment of my Dad's love, it was always an anxious moment. I liked the chocolate, but I hated what was happening around the ceremony. I would often feel a sense of being deprived of love, when my piece was not as big as the others. I felt like there wasn't enough simple love, celebration, or laughter in our home. At my grandmother's house suddenly I was the center of attention and I could eat however I liked. Overnight, my diet went crazy. I ate pasta every single night, and a lot of it. I gained twenty pounds in three months, and nobody did anything about it besides speak about my change in hormones. They just let me blow up like a balloon. I grew more and more miserable, and found refuge in more food, creating a vicious circle.

So, who was the enemy of whom?

I have abused you, a lot, with food, sugar, and diet pills that those dangerous doctors gave you, and like a silly goose I trusted them so much. I remember one doctor who was attracted to me after I reached my weight-loss goal because I was slender again and very beautiful. He was very handsome, and I felt attracted to him as well, but it paralyzed me. I was only eighteen, and he was married, so I freaked out when he asked me to sleep with him. I went home and gained ten pounds in one week as an instinctive way to say no. That was the beginning of a long pattern of saying no to men by gaining weight. Today it is the way to say no to myself as well. If by getting slender I don't get what I hoped I would get, namely love, or if men pursue me, asking me to sleep with them instead of loving me first, I sabotage myself by getting fat.

Oh my aching body, how betrayed I feel by you. Is the anger toward you, or is it toward them: Nado, my husband, all the others . . . You hurt right now. Am I hurting you instead of screaming at them . . . or is it my fault for allowing it to be done to me? The search is intense and you are hurting more and more . . . all over. What am I doing wrong? Even being in bed does not stop the pain, the shortness of breath. You are becoming ugly and I hate you right now. I am so afraid that if I get ugly Nado will not hold my hand . . . and then I will die. I am so far from loving you. I need someone to teach me how. I would love to love you, but like always, my love seems so conditional. Do I have to surrender, and let you take the lead? Do I have to discover what it is to be female with you too? I'm scared, and I don't trust you, and I don't trust myself with the agreements I make with you, because I always break them. I want to escape, and you keep me here with the pain. Where can I go besides facing it, feeling it, discovering all the dimensions of it and the madness connected with it? You are dying, dear body, and I don't know what to do. Tell me what to do!

In reality, blaming my body was a tricky way to avoid facing all the self-abuse I had inflicted on it over the years. If I blamed my body, or the circumstances of my life, or Nado, then I could play the role of the victim and escape taking personal responsibility. The anger I was feeling was actually more a form of resistance than of true anger because I was not yet willing to be accountable for my situation. I wanted only to blame and feel righteous. I was pointing the finger outside of myself as a way to avoid looking inside and facing myself.

It was also partly due to my fear of expressing anger. I have always been afraid of real anger, and have repressed it most of my life. I was always afraid that if I let go of control, I would be like a bottomless volcano erupting. I also feared that the explosion would hurt the people around me, and that I would end up alone.

5

Meeting
My Demons

IN MY CHILDHOOD, whenever anger was directed at me, I withdrew into a feeling of total helplessness. Violence especially would terrify me, and I would do anything to escape it. I would shut down and become totally numb. I would isolate from my family, feeling as if I were living in the "wrong house" and judging human beings as very strange. Later in life, I learned other tools of escape, like closing my eyes and doing a pretend "meditation," hoping that the angry person would go away.

I now know that the healthiest way to release anger is to express it outwardly, in a liberating way, without blaming others. For example, shouting "Fuck you!" and beating a pillow, or screaming wildly in front of the ocean. This releases the repressed energy that literally makes us sick. By emptying ourselves as much as possible, we make room for healing energy to move through us. When anger is appropriately channeled, it can serve us. It can assist us in setting up healthy boundaries and protecting ourselves from abuse. This is not done by screaming at the people in our life, but by first releasing the repressed energy on our own. This creates the opportunity to communicate our hurt feelings in an appropriate and honest manner.

Many of my spiritual teachers and therapists throughout the years had consistently told me, "Niro, one day you will have to reach the bottom of your anger," and one day I did. Life in all of its abundance presented me with the perfect circumstances.

When Nado first received the results of his test from the ashram, and we were hoping that the results were a mistake, we became very close again for a few weeks. All my resentment disappeared, and I vowed that we would tackle this challenge together until the very end. After we both tested HIV-positive, Nado withdrew and began avoiding me again. I was devastated to discover that, even in a time like this, we could not find a way to communicate and support each other. Months later he confessed that because he had felt so guilty at the time, it had been easier for him to accept my anger and blame than to receive my love and support. Losing my connection with Nado again hurt so much that my desire for living diminished greatly and I began to welcome the onset of more severe symptoms. A dangerous voice within me would whisper, "Let's get this over with quickly. Life is too disappointing."

In his own way Nado was trying to stay connected with me, but his attempts only made things worse. He was in a relationship with a man whom he referred to as his friend, but it was obvious that they were more than just friends. In an effort to integrate his two lives, Nado would invite his friend home in the hope that the two of us would grow to like each other. Could he not see that he was asking too much of me? I finally reached my limit one day while Nado was playing tennis with his friend. I could no longer restrain my anger and repulsion and I ordered them both to leave. All of my repressed judgments about homosexuality oozed out of me like poison. I really wanted to hurt Nado. I wanted to humiliate him in front of his "friend" and make him understand how misused I felt. In fact, I wanted him to see the loneliness and abandonment I felt while watching him have fun without me.

Losing Nado, being ostracized by my spiritual family, and having a terrifying disease was all too much to bear. Life no longer seemed worth living. My spiritual teachers had taught me to accept life as it comes, but this was too much to accept. How much more could I be asked to withstand? I had to draw the line somewhere, didn't I? Then, almost in answer to my innocent inquiry, that old familiar voice of my inner judge would come, like a punisher delighting in her vengeance. She would tell me how much I deserved my misfortunes as punishment for all my wrongdoings, and especially for having pretended that I did not see these misdeeds as I was doing them. Then the complainer in me would grumble that this was not the way she wanted to live her life, and continuously compare it to how it should be.

Whenever I listened to those negative inner voices, I felt shame, resentment, and a desire for vengeance. Those voices also generated a sense of urgency and panic, and a need to escape. When I didn't let those voices run me, it was easier to return to my heart. I repeatedly tried to create a new understanding between Nado and me, but to no avail. We just could not find a way to be open with each other simultaneously. We were so out of sync with each other. When I reached out to him, he would withdraw. When he reached out to me, I would blame him, so that I could feel righteous.

Because I loved Nado so dearly, I could accept on one level that he was sexually active with other men. Even though it hurt a lot, I managed to deal with it, since I was unable to compete with them. Then one day I was driving home, approaching the estate, and I saw Nado leaving in a strange car with a woman driving. Since he barely acknowledged me as they were driving away, I assumed that they were having an affair.

I couldn't take any more; something snapped inside of me. I couldn't control myself, and I became a wild animal. I had been praying for an opportunity to release the pressure of the rage repressed within me, and this was it. I had expected it to be a great thunderstorm, but I had no idea it would be a hurricane. I stormed into Nado's private cottage, barged into his bedroom, and systematically began destroying everything that had anything to do with us. I shredded books, demolished tapes, and violently smashed crystals on the floor. I let myself lose control, justified by my feelings of being betrayed.

When my first wave of anger subsided, I felt guilty for behaving so "insanely." Filled with shame, I left his cottage. Suddenly I stopped and looked up at the stars. My heart was pounding. I felt so alive, so warm and passionate. I realized that there was much more anger inside of me, ready to explode. This was the place where I had always repressed my natural flow of energy. But now I felt a second wave rising in me. I ran back to the cottage and let myself express my rage until I fell on my knees feeling completely empty. In that instant I experienced one of the most exquisite moments of bliss I can remember.

The next day when I saw Nado again, he explained to me that the woman I saw with him was one of his poetry students who was driving him to class. When he discovered his room was totally ransacked he commented with a loving smile, "I am so glad you finally went there." I was too. We held each other and were united again. In the clarity of that moment we both understood why we were together on this mysterious adventure called life and how many doors we were opening for each other. We realized that because we were constantly challenging each other by "pushing each other's buttons," we were keeping each other aware of the areas of our lives that we needed to work on. This supported us in continuing to discover who we were in relation to each other, to our disease, and to life.

As the days passed, I became more and more frustrated about how unfair life seemed to be. I was ready to give up. I was living in that dangerous place of "either-or." Somewhere in my subconscious mind I held the belief that no matter what I did, it would not produce the promised results, so what was the point of continuing? In search of an answer I examined my childhood, to see what decision this belief may have been based on. Then I remembered.

When I was ten years old, my parents had promised to send me to summer camp if I received good grades in school. For the entire school year I really worked hard and earned a total average of 98 percent. My teacher mentioned that I really deserved 100 percent, but said she could not write that on a report card. When it came time to go to camp, my parents reneged on their part of the bargain, and did not allow me to go.

I felt cheated and betrayed. From that moment on, I lost trust in my parents and despised them for not keeping their word. The set of beliefs I adopted about life on that day, such as "People can't be trusted" and "Life won't give me what I deserve," still impact my life today. I rarely trust authority figures and I am always wary of being used by people, especially in relationships. It was a very uncomfortable step, finally to acknowledge that I did not trust most people, especially my life partners. Because I rarely trusted that they would fulfill the promises they made to me, I would usually take over and fulfill them myself, being the "independent woman" that I am; yet at the same time I would resent them for not taking care of me. I can now see how I would sabotage any opportunity to receive, because I usually didn't give my partners the chance to give to me in the first place.

That incident with my parents created a series of strong filters that colored the way I perceived life. Since I was now challenged by a life-threatening illness, and my whole life seemed to be caving in, I realized it was finally time to let go of the old resentment and blame I was still holding on to from an event that happened over thirty years ago. I was finally willing to see that those beliefs needed to be examined, and that perhaps they were no longer appropriate in my life as an adult.

Today, I can finally accept what happened and my response to it. I can see that my parents were not aware of the impact that the incident had on me, and never intended to hurt me. In fact, they were doing their best to take care of me. Those old beliefs I had been carrying were no longer serving me. I accepted that the memories would always be there, but realized that they hurt me only because I kept returning to them as a way of justifying the mechanism of today's reactions. I deliberately chose to use my precious life force to empower myself rather than feed the victim in me.

It was only when I was willing to accept the past, and let go, for at least a few moments, of the decisions I had made as a child, that I had glimpses of the fact that my view of life was not actually real. It was a product of those childhood vows ("I will never let someone hurt me like that! I will never tell the truth! I will never love, it hurts too much!") that created the filters through which I perceive "reality."

In those moments of clarity I was able to embrace the perfection of life itself, and to be grateful for the constant opportunities it provides. Ultimately it was and is my choice whether or not to keep feeding that self-righteous voice within me, which I call the controller.

The controller is the part of me that would rather die than not get what she wants. She tries to control everything, at any price. She was the one who demanded closeness and intimacy from Nado, but could not be open to what was actually happening between us. She was able to justify her action and attitude from here to the end of time, with absolutely no humility, compassion, or love toward Nado or myself. She literally believed she needed the love and approval of others in order to survive, yet she was totally blind to the impossibility of the fulfillment of her request because even I was not willing to accept what was happening. That belief more than any other was draining most of my energy and making me sick. It kept me feeling hopeless, miserable, and trapped.

That belief, which at the time I considered my reality, also originated from my childhood conditioning and was based on another very basic conclusion made at a very early age. When we are born, we are helpless beings depending solely on our parents for survival. They are the source of our food, shelter, comfort, and, most importantly, love. During these early years, because we don't yet understand the spoken language fully, we learn from our parents by modeling ourselves after them. We sense whether they approve of our behavior or not. Approval feels like love, and disapproval feels like the removal of love. Our parents' approval is of the utmost importance to us, for without it we fear that they will stop taking care of us and abandon us. Since we are helpless as infants, and unable to take care of ourselves, if we were to be abandoned we would literally die. This basic fear is very present in almost all of our subconscious programming. It becomes more complex and sophisticated, embellished by the poetry of romance, as we get older, but it still originates from the conditioning of the helpless infant within us, who literally believes she needs to be taken care of by someone (Mommy, Daddy, or a surrogate) to survive. Because of this she continually confuses love with approval.

While I was in that unhealthy relationship with Nado, I never even questioned the validity of needing someone else's love to "survive." It definitely appeared to be the truth, although I know now that it was only my perceived reality.

I realize today that I was doing what I see so many of us do. I was using all of my training, as well as developing new tools, to keep those old beliefs alive. I would even go so far as to pretend that I wanted to change, when in reality I was not very interested in changing. Even though intellectually I knew it was time to examine each belief and "voice" within my head, I was afraid of letting go of my old conditioning. I was afraid I would "disappear" if I were to really examine who I thought I was, and be willing to let go of my "identity" in the process.

Occasionally, when I was totally exhausted, and no longer had the energy to resist, blame, or complain, the voice of my intuitive healer would guide me toward surrender. She reminded me that I was in charge of my life and that it was time to take responsibility for what I knew inside of me. She encouraged me to move beyond my conditioning with all its judgment and shame, and to stop trying to control the circumstances. My inner healer invited me simply to see that there was no need to resist any longer, and that it was time to move on. Somewhere deep within me I knew that it was time to let go, and to explore what I knew in my soul.

At that time in my life, I could not see the immense gift that I was receiving. Because my energy was geared toward resistance, I perceived everything that was happening as if it were an indication of my life falling apart, yet in actuality it was my wake-up call. It was the universe's way of telling me that it was time to wake up and take responsibility for my life. Unfortunately, I was not ready for such a rude awakening. I wanted to roll over and go back to sleep, hoping that the nightmare would go away. Even though my life seemed to be falling apart as the old was dying, I resisted the birth of the new simply because I was unaware of what I was doing.

6

The Healing Yes

AFTER LIVING in the contraction of "hell," and resisting my demons for the first few weeks after my diagnosis, I stumbled across a little book whose title enticed me: *The Lazy Man's Guide to Enlightenment,* by Taddeus Golas. I opened it, and there on the final page was the sentence, "When you learn to love hell, you will be in heaven." That sentence opened my eyes to what I already intuitively knew. Accept the moment the way it is, and embrace life the way it unfolds.

In that instant, I felt complete and total alignment with my self and my life for a few exquisite seconds. In that moment I could accept hell, since I was living in it, but surprisingly I discovered that it was not as easy to love heaven. Somewhere in my conditioning I believed that I did not deserve it, and that I wasn't worthy of it. I believe this was a major source of my disease.

I realized that when it came to taking care of my kids it was easy to access the samurai fighter inside of me, but when it came to myself, especially in terms of my diagnosis, I was really lost. Facing the fact that I could die soon was more than a "fight" for me. I did not know how to deal with it, and the samurai within me, usually full of energy to create solutions in the face of adversity, was not available.

As a therapist, I have worked with many people who, when they received their diagnosis, immediately vowed to fight it. Unlike them, I did not know how to feel. In fact, I realize now, I did not know how to live. Like many of us, I lived my life according to a series of determinations of what made me feel good or bad, and what was comfortable versus what was a struggle. I was just surviving, and what I considered happiness was basically the avoidance of problems and pain.

As I became aware of the absence of my fighting spirit, it seemed as if my only option was to yield completely into my feminine energy of acceptance. I was at the crossroads of finally accepting the fact that I had a deadly virus in my body. I had bought into the myth that AIDS was one-hundred-percent fatal and highly contagious, as was almost universally believed at the time.

The fact that I could infect others was actually the most horrible aspect of having the disease. At that time I was as neurotic as the masses. I was afraid that the virus might be contagious by drinking from the same cup, or sharing the same toilet seat. The fact that I could possibly infect my children was unbearable. I remember thinking that if someone had to pay for my "mistakes" it would be me, but definitely not my children. All of those ingredients of fear boiled in my head as in a pressure cooker, and I felt as if I were literally going mad.

I was so overwhelmed that I forgot all of my tools and training, and denied what my intuition was telling me. I probably just needed someone to remind me to trust my intuition. That is why I believe so strongly in workshops and support groups. They are a place where we can remind each other that we have the answers inside of us. We just need to take the time to be quiet with ourselves, to be open and available and listen.

Fortunately I was living on the beach. I had only to glance out the window to see the eternal dance of the ocean waves. Ebb and flow. In and out. Day and night. No matter how I was feeling, the waves were always dancing their dance, participating in the natural cycle of life. The majesty of the waves and the purity of the deserted winter beach spoke directly to my heart with its tender poetry. They did not change whether I was miserable or blissful. They were always there, available for me to watch, appreciate, and be nourished by. I was sad for having taken them for granted during my resentful moods. How could I have forgotten to take the time to receive them and let my heart dance in communion with them for at least a few moments each day?

The ocean was like my lover, and taught me the natural cycle of expansion and contraction. As I watched the tide approach and withdraw, it slowly dawned on me like the sun peeking out over the ocean's horizon that the cycle of expansion and contraction was happening inside of me as well. I realized that my entire being and the entire life cycle on this planet responds to this natural rhythm, this continuous pulse of contraction and expansion. Inhale-exhale, day-night, summer-winter, birth-death. It is an inevitable cycle that we can resist but we cannot change.

The ocean would guide me with its gentle fidelity, opening my eyes to the simple beauty of the now. In each precious moment of communion, the poison of my life was purified. Judging, comparing, and demanding that things be different were no longer important. I felt that I was in a state of expansion in which my awareness grew wider and was no longer exclusively focused on my problems. I was able to appreciate the beauty and simplicity of the gift of being alive.

My body immediately responded to my shift in awareness by releasing the tension it had been holding for so long. It felt like a deep "aaaah." I could breathe again. I felt so much lighter as I let myself revel in the simple yet magnificent dance of the ocean waves. Then my judgmental mind would come rushing in like the surf, questioning how I could possibly be blissful when there were so many reasons why I should feel miserable. Each time I would surrender and open myself again to the expansion of the moment, my mind would return with its judgments about how terrible my life was and I would fall into a state of contraction. My body would become tense again, like a knot, and ache all over. My breathing would be shallow, and I would pace around the house, unable to relax.

Because my body's response to my mind's judgments was so strong, I did not realize that I had a choice. If I had only recognized that fear and acceptance are just another expression of the dance between contraction and expansion, I could have said yes to the cycle, allowing the energy to flow naturally between the opposite extremes. Like most of us, I was attached to the feeling of expansion, and feared the feeling of contraction. Therefore I resisted the natural cycle of contraction and expansion. Also, in a strange way, feeling miserable and dwelling on my low self-esteem felt so familiar that it was usually easier to remain in a state of contraction and fear.

I was using my energy to say no to life, even though this was completely contrary to everything I had learned as a disciple. It was the complete opposite of what I knew was "right" on an intellectual level. Now that life was offering me the opportunity to really experience the lesson, I resisted. Then I realized I was trusting the strength of resistance and control, and distrusting the power of acceptance. Before I could really say yes to life, with its myriad of challenges, I had to accept my negative feelings.

I slowly learned to say yes to my feelings of contraction by taking long walks on the beach. The ocean accepted me exactly as I was in the moment without caring whether I was feeling contraction or expansion. I eventually learned to match that acceptance within myself. Looking back, I realize that accepting the contraction of my mind was a doorway to experiencing the expansion of my soul.

To say yes to my contraction, I had to accept my anger, fear, guilt, and shame. I began to say yes to it all, since I could no longer say no. That's where I was at that moment. There was nothing I could do to change. I was pissed off about having this fucking disease. I was angry that Nado rejected me. I felt guilty about dying so early and leaving my children on their own. I was afraid of suffering and ending up as a helpless vegetable. I was in the throes of darkness. When I acknowledged and accepted what I was truly feeling, the dam inside of me finally burst open. Waves of emotion flooded out, clearing the passage for healing and for the new to come in.

It is vitally important that we learn to respect this passage. When we are overwhelmed by the circumstances of life, and feel we have reached our limit, we become open to the possibility of healing. When I work with clients who express that they've had enough, and they can't take any more, I always think, "Hallelujah, now the work can really begin."

It is through this painful passage of surrendering control that we find ourselves on the other side of darkness, feeling naked and vulnerable, like a brand-new baby. In this moment we are reborn with the opportunity to rediscover the mystery of life and begin living from a totally different perspective. This creates the opening for miracles to happen.

By saying yes to my anger and despair, and giving myself permission to feel my feelings, I accepted the frightened and doubting part of myself, along with the confident and knowing part. Up until that point I had always tried to be strong and to protect my loved ones. I had had to control my response to life, denying that my feelings even existed. In a word, I was trying to be superwoman. It was simply time to accept that underneath it all I was vulnerable and needed to be taken care of as well.

Learning to be true to myself, since there was no more time for lies, was a major turning point for me. I finally dropped the demands and expectations I had of myself to be someone I was not. The someone I was trying to be was a product of all the roles I had learned how to play in the attempt to please my parents, my teachers, my children, and my lovers based on years of conditioning. It was finally time to journey within and discover who I was behind all the masks. This was the beginning of my healing journey, one which I had to embark on alone.

My two children had moved to San Diego. I had chosen not to tell them about my diagnosis. I was afraid that, had they known, they would have changed their plans and stayed with me. I could easily have indulged the victim in me, using the drama of my disease to manipulate them to stay with me, but I wanted them to learn how to fly on their own. It was urgent now. That was more important than to have them stand by and watch me die. It was not easy to let them go, because at the time I had no idea whether we would ever live together again. Today I value each day we have together and appreciate the fact that they both enjoy spending time with me, not out of a sense of duty but because they choose to be with me.

In January 1986, because Nado and I were in the process of separating, we were seeing each other less and less frequently. He did not share with me what was happening with him in regard to his physical health, and tended to stay away for long periods. I was finally beginning to stand up for myself and for what I wanted, even though I may have had to bark and bite in the beginning. It was not always easy simply to communicate what I needed. Because I valued my solitude, I withdrew from my friends. I knew I had to be alone to discover what it meant to let go and surrender.

The pain of my physical symptoms and my resistance to them had been growing stronger every day and there seemed to be no way out. I knew that complaining about life and criticizing myself and the people around me only made matters worse. I could no longer continue living in denial and resistance; eventually I would have to acknowledge the fact that I would die from this disease. Yet it was not something I could discuss with anyone at the time. Although I felt that I was finally approaching a place of sanity regarding my condition, I knew that the people around me would consider it madness. Surrendering to death is something our society regards as unacceptable.

I began to examine the extent of my subconscious programming about death. While I was growing up, death had been presented as something to avoid, and I perceived it as ugly and scary. It was something we rarely talked about, and now that it was time for me to face the reality of it, I realized I had no concept of it.

The few experiences I had of terminal illness and death had not been directly connected with my own life. They had always been incidents involving the life and death of others. Even though most of them had been beloved friends and family members, it still had not been happening directly to me; I had been merely a witness to their transition from this life to the next. For example, when my father died a few years ago, the cold, embalmed corpse lying in the open casket was in such contrast with the vibrant, strong man I cherished, that I observed it with total detachment. I remember thinking that it was like watching the multicolored leaves fall to the ground in autumn. It was simply a different season in the journey of a man's life. Even though I felt sad at my own loss, I was very happy for him.

Yet now I was dying of AIDS, and somehow that seemed different.

There were times when my imminent death felt like a welcome relief from a life of pain and rejection. I felt sorry for myself and figured that, since I never got what I really wanted anyway, dying would be a great escape. I was so lost in self-pity that I didn't even consider the impact of my death on my loved ones who remained behind. Then, after I reached a certain level of weariness regarding my resentment, resistance, and denial, the reality of the disease touched me in a brand-new way. I had to make a quantum leap in personal honesty to accept that there was a killer retrovirus in my body, and that the odds were I would die soon. The moments of surrender happened sporadically and were extremely fragile. They seemed to happen by "accident," when I was too exhausted to keep complaining about the way things were.

That was the turning point of surrender. I finally said yes to my condition as a part of me. Up until that point it had been much easier to keep the illusion of separation between myself and the "enemy," in the hope that maybe it would disappear as mysteriously as it had appeared. When I honestly embraced the fact that my immune system was slowly failing me, and that I would die in eighteen months or less, the illusion of living forever, like a veil, was suddenly ripped off of my face. Yet even while I was lost in a whirlwind of fear, a quiet almost imperceptible voice reminded me, "Stay open. This experience has value. Learn from what is happening now." I knew that once I surrendered to the truth then my life would drastically change. No longer could I take tomorrow for granted.

I remember sitting at the kitchen table with a calendar, counting the 492 days I still had left if I was lucky. When I really got it in my guts that each day that passed would never return, something shifted inside of me. Suddenly each day was precious to me. It was not an intellectual understanding, it was an actual experience of each moment as sacred. I could not waste even one. This realization totally transformed the way I responded to life. I burst into seeing the fullness of each moment, and I embraced each with an open heart.

Denial, resistance, and control disappeared and were replaced with an inner strength that had not been available to me before. In that moment of surrender, the fog lifted on all the fragmented aspects of my personality, which had been fighting amongst themselves. I could recognize all my subpersonalities and their conflicts—my judgmental self was battling with the fragmented part of me that was in denial. The resistant part of me was in conflict with the mask of the people-pleaser. The controller was trying to take charge of them all. When I looked deeper behind all the masks I discovered a vulnerable little girl who was terrified of dying and who was desperately looking for someone or something to protect her.

In the beginning, the concept of surrender was a very frightening one. I had always understood surrender to be the result of a power struggle, with a winner and a loser. Because I had been approaching the disease as an external source of power over my body, the idea of surrendering magnified my fear of suffering and death. Whenever I introduce the concept of surrender to my clients, they often understand it as abandoning the fight, and they usually try to avoid it at any cost. Often they believe that if they were to surrender to the truth that they have a disease, then they would be giving power to it. The truth is, when we deny or resist something out of fear, we give our power away to fear. When we accept it as the truth, we take our power back.

Surrender does not mean giving our power away. Surrender is the path of the master and of the healer. It is saying yes to life and accepting what is so. Giving our power away is the path of the victim and of the child survivor. It is saying no to life and resisting it as it unfolds. We never actually give our power away, we simply hope to have things our own way, and we resent it when we don't. Falling into the trap of believing that we gave our power away is simply a sophisticated way to enable ourselves to complain that life didn't turn out the way we wanted.

Surrender is the simplest yet most grandiose state that a human being can reach. It is accepting things exactly the way they are in the present moment, with no past and no future. It is beyond judgment. In our daily lives we constantly operate from a critical evaluation: We say, this is good, it gives me pleasure—or we fall into the opposite, saying, this is bad, it creates pain. When was the last time you stopped to reevaluate your judgments and beliefs before acting from them? Rarely had I even considered it, yet now that I was facing my imminent death, I questioned everything. I wanted finally to discover who I was before I left this body and this life.

It was an intense beginning. I realized that I knew very little about who Niro was. I knew a lot about her past, and the personality she had created to survive. I was intimate with her mistakes, her regrets, her dreams and fantasies. I knew her reactions, but I didn't know who she really was in this moment. My lifelong dreams of world travel, and of being taken care of by the perfect partner, just fell away when I let go of my future plans. There was no more time to waste dreaming of what would be, or regretting what didn't happen. I was acutely aware that I had a finite number of days remaining on this earth (as we all do), and chose to reprioritize my life accordingly. The first thing I did was dispense with the superficial social activities that had consumed much of my time. I no longer cared about what was the "right" thing to do.

Healing energy became available to me because I was living with acceptance. Acceptance leads to forgiveness, which is an important stepping-stone to healing. Like healing, forgiveness is an allowing and not a doing. It is impossible to force forgiveness. It is the natural flowering of the seeds of surrender. For me, forgiveness happened spontaneously in the moment and became an open door to love for myself and others.

Love is the most important healing energy. It is all you need to make miracles happen. Old resentments, about events like the time my mother would not allow me to go to summer camp, just fell away in that higher energy. They were no longer important. I no longer needed to cling to them as a part of my identity, which had been built on so much unfinished business.

In the healing process, as in life itself, forgiveness means being willing to drop the past and live in the present. It is the bridge between finishing with old memories—perhaps resolving them, perhaps not—and being willing to let them go. Forgiveness is a very important step to take in learning to live in the present. It is accepting that the past is the past, that we cannot change it. All we can do is to choose to finish with the memories.

Through forgiveness I realized that, although I could not change the past, I could change the effect it had on the present. For example, if I were to judge my past actions as the source of my disease, it would create intense guilt (contraction). But with forgiveness comes freedom from judgment, and liberation from guilt. Through acceptance I experienced true freedom for the first time ever.

Acceptance created expansion and opened my heart to life as it was presented to me. I simply surrendered unconditionally, without any expectation. I wasn't bartering for more time, or a second chance; I just said yes to whatever was happening and continued with my daily chores. Even though the pain and discomfort of my body did not go away, my spirit was dancing with tremendous joy and the love of life. I was learning to accept the dance between contraction and expansion, and discovering what it meant to exist in the space between them.

Because I finally accepted the unacceptable, I was able to detach from my worries and concerns. I experienced life from a different perspective. Instead of becoming more terrified and contracted by death, I felt a deep sense of release and expansion. I embarked on a very powerful journey of questioning, of choices, of doubt and of fear. It was a journey from merely surviving on automatic pilot to consciously living the gift of life in all its glory.

As I surrendered to life itself, I was able to become more detached from the many stressful details that had been cluttering it. Letting go of the importance I had placed on them created a fresh ease which I had been lacking for what seemed like forever. I felt so alive, and so real in my feelings. I watched my emotions as they constantly changed, like the seasons. I accepted them all, the fear as well as the joy, without judging them as good or bad. As with the ocean, nothing was static inside or outside of me. I was a part of the ongoing rhythm of life. What the Chinese call the Tao or "the way." More and more I let go and felt my place in life's miraculous flow.

7

Living
with Integrity

I WAS VERY SURPRISED that the extremely self-centered part of me (which I call the indulger) did not take over my life and run wild. I could have indulged my sweet tooth, stuffing myself with chocolate, ice cream, and all kinds of other fattening goodies, or gone on a shopping spree, loading my credit cards to the max, or just laid around in bed all day doing nothing. I could have totally given up and let go of any kind of discipline—because, as the indulger believed, "Since I'm gonna die nothing really matters." It was so strange that the voice of indulgence, which had always rationalized about starting that diet tomorrow, or postponing exercise today, did not show up. That voice of a million excuses had rarely been silent, except for the few times when I was very happy and felt loved.

I began to identify those very different parts of myself. On the one side was the indulger or victim, whose main thrust is fear and survival; on the other side was the voice of integrity, the healer, whose path is one of self-mastery and beingness. Indulgence created a false sense of expansion in me because my desires were temporarily satisfied, but ultimately it led to discomfort and contraction. On the other hand, integrity created an organic sense of expansion, not from doing anything in particular, but from being true to myself. Still, it was difficult to stay with my integrity because it was so easy to slip into indulgence. It often demanded extreme self-discipline to say no to my indulgence and say yes to what I knew was best for me.

I could not escape noticing how much my symptoms worsened when I went into the "poor me" pattern, so I created a very simple discipline to avoid indulging the "victim" in me. Each day, I committed myself to accomplishing three things, regardless of how badly I felt. In fact, I would not go to bed until they were completed. The three tasks might be balancing my checkbook, sewing on a missing button, and giving myself a manicure. Because I knew the power of my indulger, I was careful not to challenge myself too much; I chose goals that I knew I could achieve. I set myself up to win, and to go to bed with the satisfying sense of having accomplished something valuable. Most importantly of all, I kept my word with myself. It was very expansive and healing to look at my life and feel that things were in order. Accomplishing my three daily goals gave me that feeling, and as a result the quality of my sleep each night was much more nourishing. I also made a point to maintain an impeccable appearance. I did not want to look the part of a sick person at this early stage.

Living a disciplined lifestyle was a new experience for me. I no longer imposed impossible challenges on myself, only to become discouraged when I was unable to fulfill them. I practiced keeping my word with myself, one step at a time. It was like working a muscle that has not exercised in a long time. In the beginning, it is weak and shaky. Practice is needed, and mistakes happen. The newness of the experience makes it clumsy and sore. Yet with time and perseverance, the muscle grows stronger and more alive, a vital part of the body.

My indulgence had been endlessly sabotaging me, not only in terms of my physical health, but also in the quality of my relationship with Nado. At times it had also affected my attitude toward my children and my job. Following my diagnosis, my constant complaining and my need to control and resist continued to disempower me. Finally I had had enough. It was time to stop indulging, time to discover what it was to be honest with myself, take full responsibility for my actions, and live with that integrity.

For years, I had thought of "integrity" as synonymous with "self-criticism." Every time someone would mention my integrity, it was basically to criticize me for my lack of it. So the idea of integrity and the feeling of being chastised, by both myself and others, always seemed to be intertwined.

I had first begun to learn how to take honest responsibility for my life when I was in the est Guest Seminar Leader program, which was very demanding. In order to find the time to keep all my commitments, I literally did not sleep several nights a week. Although I usually overextended myself, it was wonderful to keep my word, not to have to lie or avoid people with whom I had broken agreements. Living honestly was extremely exhilarating, but tough on the body—so then I ended up equating honesty with stress. When I was first learning how to communicate my truth with others, my fear of rejection often created a high level of stress within me. I had no idea that it could be another way.

Now I realized that it was time to discover my own experience of what it meant to live at maximum potential, as opposed to what I had learned from others in books and seminars. I embarked on a journey to discover what integrity really meant to me. I began to understand it as a simple way of living my life. I slowed down my entire life, continually asking myself the question: "Will this action or decision support me to reach my maximum potential?" I still ask myself this question today. Whenever I lose sight of my direction in life and feel as if I'll never get back on track, I simply ask the question again to realign with myself.

As part of my exploration, I also asked myself what steps I could take that would support me in reaching my maximum potential. It was always important for me to be the best I could be, and eventually to fulfill my life's purpose, once I finally discovered what it was. Now, since I knew I would die, there was very little time. Although I was willing to die, I wanted to fulfill my purpose for being on this planet first. It was important to me that I discover my reason for being, or my "raison d'être," as they say in Belgium. I opened myself up to the question and waited patiently for the answer, in silence, not in time, since time had become my enemy.

Eventually an even more basic question arose, and I asked myself, What exactly was my maximum potential? Again I simply let go and stayed open to receive the answer, without trying to figure it out. For me, the exploration of that dance between the question and the answer is one of the greatest motivations to be alive. By simply letting myself bathe in the silence of this question, without all my preconceived conclusions, the answer eventually surfaced from deep inside of me. My maximum potential is living with love for myself and others, and creating love and beauty all around me like an endless circle . . . a dance of giving and receiving.

I realize now that prior to my diagnosis I was living a life that mostly went against my own nature, while I was pretending that it was the way I wanted to live. I had kept experimenting with various lifestyles, from housewife to jet-setter to spiritual disciple, in search of the one that corresponded to my true nature.

The pretense that life was fine had created such an enormous stress on my system that it provided a perfect fertile ground for disease to erupt from. My immune system was so weakened by this self-denial, and by a deep sense of unworthiness, that it was not able to respond effectively to the invasion of the HIV infection.

By living my life according to my own needs instead of constantly trying to please others as I had been conditioned to do, I experienced a glimpse of what it felt like to "put myself on the top of the list." I began to stand up for myself and what my needs were, in spite of the fact that many of my friends and relatives could not understand my "strange behavior." It was finally time to rediscover what Niro genuinely wanted, which was extremely frightening. All of my conditioning stood in the way. I still have difficulty with the issue of serving versus pleasing, especially in romantic relationships. My conditioning is so strong, and the desire to be liked and accepted so powerful, that it demanded a strong effort for me to stay true to what felt right to me. At the beginning of my healing journey, I was not cognizant of the difference between serving others and trying to please others. I know now that there is a huge qualitative difference. The desire to serve others comes from an overflow of the heart, where giving becomes receiving; trying to please others comes from a desperate need for approval in hopes that we won't be rejected and hurt.

Since I had very little time left to bother with trying to please the world, I put myself on the top of the list. Up until that point I had believed that if I put myself first, I would be putting others down, and I did not want to be selfish. I now see that this "self-ishness" was a key ingredient to my healing. Putting myself on the top of the list was a real challenge, because I had learned that in order to love others I had to put myself down. Although this was not taught outright, it was subtly implied in my religious upbring-ing. It came from a Catholic tradition of suffering and repression where martyrs are canonized as saints. Ironically, the more I put myself down, the less available I was to truly love another. I had always believed that if I gave a certain amount to someone, then I should receive a certain amount back from them. Suddenly, once I put myself on the top of the list, loving others became a direct reflection of loving myself. I gave up trying to please everyone, and simply gave from the simplicity of my heart.

When I took the risk to stand up for myself and go for what I long for, many of my friends felt I was behaving like a spoiled, capricious brat. Some friendships disappeared, while others deep-ened. Even though I made lots of mistakes along the way, putting myself on the top of the list helped prioritize my life. The things that were important, like loving relationships with my family and friends, stayed, and what was superfluous, like social acquaintan-ces, fell away.

I was finally learning how to establish my boundaries. In fact, my inability to establish boundaries had been a major emotional factor contributing to my disease. My sense of shame about not living up to the standards imposed on me by my parents had made me susceptible to abuse from others. So as part of my search for my maximum potential I needed to discover what my personal bound-aries were in relation to the people in my life.

For example, Nado would frequently disappear into the city for two or three days, without telling me where he was going or when he would return, leaving me to take care of his chores. Upon his return he would withdraw from me, avoiding any eye contact, as if he were ashamed by his behavior. There were times when he would return from his journey into darkness appearing so desperate and lost that all I wanted to do was hold him and tell him, "It's all right, baby, you're gonna be fine," but he would never allow me to. I could feel the pain of his guilt and his struggle with his sexual identity and addiction. Unfortunately, any dialogue concerning these issues was impossible.

It eventually became too much. Not only did I have to deal with my own pain and my own approaching death, but I had to deal with the unspoken torment of my estranged lover, who refused to open up to me. His mysterious disappearances became so unbearable that I would wake up in the middle of the night, delirious from the night sweats, screaming his name in a panic.

Because our life circumstances were so confrontational in and of themselves, we would do just about anything to avoid taking on any more conflict. Although clinging to each other may have appeared to be the most convenient solution at the time, it only ended up feeding our loneliness and adding to the resentment we felt toward each other.

Finally, in a therapy session with one of my colleagues, I saw clearly that I did not want to live the last months of my life feeling as I did. Up until that session, it never occurred to me that I had the right to establish boundaries and say, "No more, this hurts too much. It is killing me more than the disease itself." I went home that day after the session and finally asked Nado to pack his bag and leave. He looked at me silently for a moment, and then walked away. Moments later, I went upstairs to my bedroom and discovered a beautiful dusty-rose coat hanging in front of my closet with a love note from Nado. I felt horrible. The timing seemed so off, but then, the timing always seemed off when it came to respecting my boundaries.

Finally standing up for myself and asking Nado to leave, knowing that he was sicker than I, was one of the most courageous events of my life. Not only did I have to let go of the dream of us spending our lives together, but I also had to face the fact that I was not the endlessly patient and compassionate person I wanted to believe I was.

It was excruciating to watch him pack up all of his belongings. I felt so desperate, like I had failed one more time. Yet, surprisingly, the moment he left, I felt so relieved. I could breathe again. Only after his departure did I realize just how much I had denied myself during those two years with Nado. Now it was time to rediscover who I was in my solitude. I had made a choice that would empower me to grow because I had finally stopped enabling the victim in Nado as well as in myself. I could now live sanely in my solitude until my death.

Up until that point, I had been terrified of being alone. I had confused being alone with being lonely. As a teenager, I was too embarrassed to be seen taking public transportation alone and would hide in taxis instead. Now I was spending entire days by myself, meditating and taking long walks on the beach. Day by day, I was timidly discovering how much I truly did love myself. Meditation was the key to that discovery. It was the beginning of a real love affair with myself that still continues today.

Most of the meditations I practiced were active meditations designed by Osho to assist the modern Western man in emptying himself of all the repressed emotions that keep him from experiencing the silence within. They involved using the whole body in a vigorous and sometimes strenuous manner. Because my energy was low and my body was still fragile in the beginning, I chose the Nadabrahma meditation, the least physically demanding of them all. The Nadabrahma is based on an old Tibetan technique of humming. It is a beautiful meditation that focuses on the harmony between giving and receiving.

After meditation I felt such exquisite inner peace that I got hooked. I loved meditating because it was the way I longed to live, moment to moment, in an appreciation of the miracle of life. I was no longer judging, reacting to, or trying to change what was; I simply witnessed it. I didn't meditate in order to get something, to become healed or enlightened, but just because that was who I was in that moment. I felt so excited, and interested in life. It no longer mattered whether the nights were uncomfortable, or whether getting out of bed was a big production. That was my life at the moment, and I was saying yes to it.

Meditation assisted me in changing my tendency to dwell in the past, and worry about the future. Through meditation I learned how to live in the present moment. Not only did I sit and meditate several times a day, but everything I did became meditation. This practice is what saved my sanity.

For example, when I baked muffins I would focus my complete attention on the act of baking. Instead of dividing my awareness between baking and thinking of why I was baking, whether the muffins would taste all right, what my plans were for later, etc., I would discipline myself to observe the experience of what was happening in the present moment. I would keep asking myself the question, "What is now? I am baking muffins. My bare feet are on the floor and I can feel the cool freshness of the tiles. What is now? My hands are opening the bag of flour and pouring some into a measuring cup. What is now? My back hurts, my stomach is growling, and I feel the air in my lungs as I breathe." When I worked in the garden I focused totally on the plants and soil, tuning everything else out. When I walked on the beach I allowed the beauty and tranquility of the moment to nourish me completely. This mindful awareness kept me in the reality of the moment instead of lost in the painful "movie" of yesterday and tomorrow. It's like they say in the twelve-step recovery programs of Alcoholics Anonymous: One day at a time. I literally lived one moment at a time. It was the only way I had of dealing with the waves of tremendous fear that would wash up on the shore sporadically throughout the day. Otherwise, I would have lost my mind long before I lost my life.

I had always wanted to learn to live in the present moment, and it seemed like now was the time to develop a discipline to do that, for the sake of my sanity. I did not need a demanding discipline, but a willingness to live with mindful awareness. It was quite difficult in the beginning and required a lot of energy. The paradox lay in my wanting desperately to escape the demons of my mind, but in seeing how automatically I let them run. It was as if I had no ability to halt the train of my thoughts.

Through meditation, I discovered that thoughts had no power by themselves. I could choose to engage in them, or to bring my awareness back to my breath in the present moment. I was able to observe the constant reactions I had to my thoughts. By simply watching each thought, followed by each reaction, I slowed down the automatic thought process. This created a tiny gap between thought and reaction. Soon I could begin to choose a new response, or even no response to the thought. After a while I realized that being run by my fearful thoughts was another form of indulgence. I had a choice. It was my responsibility to start consciously choosing moment by moment.

8

My Daily
Awareness Routine

ONE DAY while meditating, I was guided by the common sense of my intuition and I created what I call my daily awareness routine. It consisted of daily meditation, healthy diet, regular exercise, long walks on the beach, and personal hygiene for my neglected body. One by one I began to utilize the tools I had learned in various workshops and had read about in countless books. This time, though, my discipline was not imposed on me from someone outside of me, but from my own inner wisdom. I was not submitting to the rules of any organization or external authority, but to my own self-empowering guidelines.

The daily awareness routine I developed was mine, and although it required effort, I felt little or no resistance to it. Accomplishing my goals was empowering, and if some rules needed to be adapted for certain circumstances, it was easy to use my creativity to adjust to whatever was appropriate. This process was always guided by my response to the question, "What do I want?" and "Will this serve me in reaching my maximum potential?"

The change in my attitude was a key ingredient in establishing my own definition of integrity. When I was following the rules "imposed" on me (even though I know I am the one who chose to be part of the organization), the rebel in me resisted, as a safeguard against being controlled and possibly hurt. Rebelling is of course a natural defense mechanism, but it is such a reactive state that it made me a prisoner of the issue I was rebelling against.

Even so, my need to belong would usually override my resistance, and I would submit to the rules. Unfortunately, I didn't follow them from the ease of surrender but from the fear of rejection. Slowly I became a victim of the system, by my own doing. That is why today I advise my students and clients to refrain from copying what I or others did, and instead to discover what resonates in them, creating what I call their own "prescription." Then everything can fall into place naturally.

Instead of succumbing to the many "should"s imposed on me by authority, I began to be motivated by self-discipline. In other words, instead of succumbing to or rebelling against external authoritarian power, I tapped into my own internal authentic power. For example, we are told we should "eat an apple a day to keep the doctor away." Often the rebel in me would disregard the wisdom of this practice as a way of still saying no to my parents or my teachers. Still getting even at forty is a bit silly, but aren't we all still rebels in a certain way? With this awareness, I chose to surrender to eating the apple. I embraced the freedom of choice that was available to me by taking an action I knew was a positive and nourishing one. Eating the apple now empowers me because I am doing it of my own free will instead of having it imposed on me.

All the energy that I formerly wasted in rebellion, and then in justification, was now liberated to help me explore the simplicity and magnificence of life itself. By not indulging the part of me that was a rebel, I learned to stop feeding the victim in me. I became aware of the connection between the rebel and the victim in me. (Boy, I did not like discovering that one.)

I practiced my daily awareness routine in an atmosphere of beauty and harmony which I created all around me. I either spent my days in solitude or with people who loved me and whom I loved dearly as well. The bliss and the peace that resulted was exhilarating. I was learning to live in simple joy. I had never really lived that way before. Joy had always been dependent on someone or something outside myself, like a romantic relationship, lots of money, designer clothes, or a magnificent house. Because my attitude was now changed, my joy required nothing more than what I already had.

One of the tools I incorporated into my daily awareness routine was the result of an "accident." This was the technique of using visualization or mental imagery. I was doing Kundalini meditation, an active meditation which involves shaking the body totally to reach a higher state of consciousness and a lighter physical density. As I was shaking to loud pulsating music that is designed specifically to facilitate the process of letting go, the electrical power went off, and the music stopped.

The silence took me by surprise and I froze. Then something very strange happened. Somehow I could see inside of my body; I literally saw my liver, my stomach, my intestines, and my other internal organs, and they looked a putrid shade of yellowish green. It lasted for only a few moments, but the impact of this experience was so strong that I had to sit and integrate what I had just seen. Shocked by what I saw, I intuitively began to use mental imagery to purify and rejuvenate my internal organs. Because I was so revolted by the horrible color, I imagined the Niagara Falls flushing away all that green stuff out of my liver and stomach. Since that time I have heard guided visualizations which involve a golden waterfall pouring down over you, but in my case I knew that only the tremendous power of Niagara Falls could do the job.

I also changed my diet to a healthier and lighter one to cleanse my body of its toxins. As I mentioned earlier, my diet was very indulgent. Although I considered myself a vegetarian, I ate very few vegetables. I may have refrained from meat, poultry, and fish, but I also refrained from almost any foods that had any nutritional value. (I daresay coffee and French bread could not be considered a well-balanced diet, even in Paris.)

The gentle reproach and concrete guidance I received from my intuition regarding my poor nutrition was extremely powerful. I began to detest the taste of chocolate, although for a while I still indulged. Some of my clients who are recovering alcoholics have shared a similar passage in their healing process. Even though they could not stand the taste or smell of alcohol they were not yet able to stop drinking. I believe that this period of disgust toward our addiction is a very important one, providing us with the opportunity to realize the full dimension and consequences of our self-destructive pattern. Ultimately it motivates us to say yes to ourselves and our maximum potential by saying no to the addiction.

When I finally listened to my inner guidance, I went to a weight-loss clinic called Health Management. I began a medically monitored liquid diet of protein powder with an egg-white base, containing a balanced intake of vitamins, minerals, glucides, and lipids. I loved it. It simplified my relationship with food. I only had to choose between vanilla and chocolate, open an envelope, and mix it with water. Food suddenly became such an unimportant part of my life. Who had time to eat anyway? My time was so precious to me.

Back then I did not consider my diet as a way to heal. Healing from AIDS was unthinkable. I chose to lose weight, to guide my body back to its natural state of health and beauty, as a way to reach my maximum potential. It was too easy to indulge in sweets and lie in bed all day. I chose not to play the "Why me?" game, complaining about the way the universe had dealt my cards. I no longer had time for that kind of indulgence. I wanted only to be the best I could be and to live at my maximum potential.

I realize now that the liquid diet served as a kind of fast to detoxify my body. I highly recommend fasts—but strictly under medical supervision—to my clients as a way of cleansing and purifying the body of its poisons. Whether it be a modified liquid diet like mine, or a juice or water fast, it is an excellent way for the body to rejuvenate.

I can't emphasize enough how important it is that a fast be supervised by a qualified professional. This is because, as the body detoxifies, there are usually adverse reactions. If your immune system is very weak, the rapid detoxification could be very brutal on the body. For me, because I was no longer polluting my body with sugar, caffeine, and other processed chemicals, my body responded with terrible gas and constipation. (I welcomed the change from months of diarrhea.) As my body continued to detoxify, my breath smelled pungent and my skin, which is our largest organ, broke out in pimples as a result of the poisons leaving through my pores. Salt baths and dry brushing (using a dry body brush on my body to rub away dead skin), as well as regular sessions of deep breathing, were some of the tools that assisted me in the detoxifying process.

Another common symptom I suffered from was intense headaches as a result of the sugar withdrawal. I also experienced occasional nausea in response to the fast. Fortunately, my nutritional counselor was able to monitor my progress and assured me that my symptoms were a normal response to fasting and not advancing symptoms of my illness. In fact, soon after I began my daily awareness routine and changed my diet, I noticed a shift in my previous physical symptoms. My diarrhea stopped and my energy became more available. I felt better than I had in a long, long time.

My household chores on the estate I managed were also included as part of my daily awareness routine. Two of my favorite duties were caring for the indoor plants and creating beautiful flower arrangements for my employer. They were nourishing connections with nature, and brought a lot of joy into my life.

I also began to exercise. In the beginning I would walk for a few minutes, and that was all I could accomplish. Yet instead of judging how pitiful it was to be in such bad shape, I praised myself for being dedicated enough to do it. Eventually I was walking four miles a day: two miles on the beach in the morning, and two miles along pastoral country roads in the evening. I also practiced t'ai chi on the beach. This not only centered me as a form of meditation but also served as a stretching and strengthening exercise for my muscles and ligaments.

I loved taking proper care of myself, and, surprisingly, it was very easy to create the time for it. The feeling of "doing the right thing" created a lightness of being that was ultimately much more fulfilling than chocolate. Each day I would awaken by six A.M., following the natural rhythm of my body. I would sit on the deck overlooking the ocean for sunrise meditation, usually the Nadabrahma, and then silently enjoy breakfast. Next I would slowly take devoted care of my body, with long showers and a thorough dry brushing of the skin. Just the ritual of caring for my body would take nearly ninety minutes.

It was very important for me to discipline myself to look good so that I could feel good about myself. I took the time to dress well, fix my hair, put on a little makeup, and look the best I could. I found that if I looked healthy, I felt healthier. Many of my clients today follow the same cue. When I visited one dear friend in the hospital, he wasn't wearing a hospital nightgown, but a pair of flashy purple pants and a lovely turquoise green T-shirt. He shared with me how important details like that were in helping him to keep his spirits high. It also gave him the sense that he was active in his healing process and not at the mercy of the sometimes demeaning atmosphere of the hospital. It is so important to respect those little details that empower us on our healing journey. It's a simple guideline, but it so often has tremendous impact. The better we look, the better we feel.

I also noticed that I had an entirely different approach to using my healing tools. Before, whenever I would learn a new tool, a new spiritual discipline, or even a diet, I used to go into it so fanatically that it would become the entire focus of my life. After a while, of course, other aspects of my life, such as my family or my job, would demand attention, and I would have to abandon everything, in a very *tout ou rieniste* ("all or nothing") way. This time, I was simply living my life, which included the use of my daily awareness tools. My tools were not my life, they were a part of it.

After four months of total discipline with my fast, I began to eat solid food again, moving into the Fit for Life diet and conscious food combining. This diet was based on the principle of natural-hygiene vegetarianism and was made popular by the Diamonds in their book *Fit for Life*. The basic principles of proper food combining originated from the theory of how digestive enzymes interact in the digestion process. Protein foods are acid-based and starch foods are alkaline-based; therefore the two do not mix well. The theory follows that if we eat a starch and protein together (like meat and potatoes, or bread and cheese), then the alkaline and acid enzymes cancel each other out. When that neutralization takes place in the stomach, the food is not digested efficiently and our digestion system does not operate as effectively as it is designed to.

Because of this, we do not receive the full nutritional value from the food we eat.

Eating solid food again was a new discovery. For the first time, I was consciously eating well to support my health as opposed to trying to lose weight. Ironically, the vain part of me was ecstatic when I dropped sixty-six pounds and once again felt beautiful and sensual. Although it was scary as well as exciting, I figured that if I was going to die, I wanted to die in a beautiful body. (Why not?) I stopped caring about the reaction of men who were attracted to me and what kind of trouble it might lead to. I gave myself permission to be a beautiful and powerful woman again and let go of any judgment or shame that may have been inhibiting me. That old fear about being attractive was still present, but this time I let myself feel it without letting it stop me. I began to discover the joy of my beauty being appreciated in an honest way, without any manipulation on my part.

I was open and available to life as it was unfolding, beyond reaction or conditioning. I simply focused on my daily awareness routine and stayed open to whatever life was offering. As my connection with the gentleness of nature, with the emptiness of silence, with the inner realms of my consciousness grew, meditation became a natural state of being, not a doing. Life became my meditation.

A simple and amazingly tender trust in my new life began to arise. By putting myself on the top of the list and practicing my daily awareness routine, I was able to let go of my need to control everyone and everything around me and be open to my life as it unfolded. I was living in the question and embracing the mystery of life, a mystery that did not demand to be solved, but only to be lived.

9

Satori

I LOVED my new life. It was very simple, and it was exactly the way I wanted it to be. Waking up in the morning had always been a precious moment for me, but now I felt such a sense of gratitude. I was utterly grateful just to be alive.

I explored my connection with the rhythm of nature in a deeper and deeper way during my long walks on the beach. Each day I aligned myself with the gentle energy of the surf. To do this I would completely focus my awareness on the waves as they crashed on the beach or on the wind as it danced on the ashen white dunes. This heightened awareness forced me to stay conscious of my present experience instead of getting lost in the thoughts of "what if" and "if only" which so often played in my head.

Meditative walks on the beach were my priorities. These daily strolls along my beloved ocean were an essential part of my daily awareness routine. I called it my Vipassana walk. Vipassana is a meditation technique which assists us in developing a state of mindful awareness by simply witnessing our thoughts and actions. Through my Vipassana walk, the ordinary experience of walking, which I had taken for granted for so many years, became an extraordinary moment of communion with myself and with the nature all around me. The technique involved slowly and consciously taking one step at a time, feeling my foot as it lifted from the soft sand, gently moving it ahead of my other foot and slowly placing it in the sand again. My concentration would be intently focused on each step, breaking it down to the many separate moments within each step. My eyes would be focused down at a forty-five-degree angle and I would walk for miles just witnessing my moment-to-moment experience of walking.

Even though it was the middle of winter, the cold weather did not deter me from taking my daily walk on the beach. I love the beach in the winter; it is so empty and nostalgic. It awakens a soft melancholy in me that I welcome, for its exquisite flavor. Those moments were like draping my naked body in silk velvet.

One cold, clear day in late March, I was bundled up tightly, taking my daily walk. The beach was covered with snow and it was utterly magical. It was not the first time that I had seen the beach like that, but on that particular day the light was different, and the sky was intensely blue. The sound of the sea was powerful yet gentle at the same time, like words of love whispered in the intimacy of lovemaking. I was alone except for a group of seagulls playing on the snow-covered sand.

As I walked along the shore, I became more and more aware of the infiniteness of the ocean. The uniqueness of each separate wave touched me while at the same time I was moved by how completely each merged with the ocean. There in front of my eyes was a perfect example of oneness. Through my appreciation of the unity between the waves and the ocean, I myself became part of the experience of merging, and felt an incredible sense of "coming home." I was deeply moved by the majestic scene in front of me. Tears of gratitude fell like raindrops returning to the sea.

As I walked, I listened to that special sound that boots make as they leave their prints in fresh snow, and enjoyed that feeling of sinking into the frosty path with each step. In that exquisite moment I was fully aware of the miracle of each breath, and of the magic of the way my bones and the muscles in my legs and ankles moved as I shifted my weight from one leg to the other. I had never experienced as much rapture and appreciation for the miracle of being alive as I felt at that instant. It was beyond bliss. It was simply a full "is-ness."

Each step was the first one and the last one. I was totally in tune with the rhythm of nature, and a deep sense of lightness was expanding from within me. I had never experienced such a sensation. It was as if the physical limitations of my body were melting away. I experienced a sense of becoming one with the vast space around me. My presence dissolved into the snow, the ocean, the sky, the birds. No longer was there a definitive separation between myself and the heat of sun, the icy cold breeze, or the roar of the surf. My breath slowed down, until it seemed like I was barely breathing. All that remained was a sensation of limitlessness.

My body stopped its pace naturally and I faced the ocean, feeling my oneness with the waves, and my arms started to rise above my head, guided by their own energy. Suddenly Osho appeared to me in a vision. Up until then, I had always held him in very high esteem, belittling myself as his humble disciple in a subtle put-down of myself. This time it was different. This time my beloved master appeared to me, on the same level as I was, and we joined in a deep embrace. I have never felt so safe and so totally a vital part of existence as I did in that sacred embrace. In a flash, I understood that the answers were not outside of me but had always been inside of me.

I was wrapped in a feeling that felt like a giant quilted comforter, a feeling that I was fine—not healed, just fine. That feeling penetrated me deeply, warming me and nourishing every one of my cells.

When we have a glimpse of the perfection of life, and when we realize that life is much bigger than our wildest dreams, our individual identity and our separate boundaries disappear. Only harmony and love remain. Love is an is-ness. It is not something we can strive to achieve. Love is our very being. It is not a feeling that is defined by the intensity generated by lust or sex. In fact, it has very little to do with that. In that moment, I understood that love is a total beingness, where there is no separation. In love, disease is embraced as part of the whole. Love is always available; we only need to get out of the way and be open to it. Love flows from complete trust, acceptance, and surrender to oneness, when the "I" disappears. Love is the ultimate merging.

It is my understanding that I experienced what is known as a satori, which is a Japanese word for "glimpse." It was a glimpse of total awareness, and for a moment I experienced an altered state of consciousness. It is a state where no questions exist, and where there is only perfection.

Following that moment of satori, I completely lost the notion of time. I don't recall very well how I got back home, and what I did after that. It all just happened perfectly. I think, if I remember correctly, that I slept for quite a long time.

Years before I probably would have jumped up and down with a great sense of achievement, but now it was clear that there was nowhere to go, and nothing to achieve. That moment was a peak, and after that I was in a valley, but in such a roaring peace, I simply let myself be transported by it. I was now totally at peace with death and even with suffering. I was really ready to accept death whenever it came, and no longer merely on an intellectual level. I also celebrated my reunion with Osho, which temporarily mitigated the loss I had been feeling because of his organization's policy prohibiting HIV-infected people from entering the ashram.

It had been a powerful experience yet at the same time a very fragile one. I was unable to speak to anyone about it, and needed time to integrate it. Even today, I am still a little shy about sharing this experience with certain people, because it is so esoteric. Even so, that glimpse of merging still affects me whenever I recall it. Sometimes just by closing my eyes I am transported back to the feeling of that mysterious experience. Merging and its opposite, rejection, have been my life's theme, and I was so grateful to have experienced the gift of total merging, and to have experienced both sides of one energy. My life could have ended at that moment and it wouldn't have mattered. I felt utterly complete. I understood that both sides had their source in the same unique light. Nothing more was needed. An unshakable trust was now rooted in me, and after that day it really no longer mattered whether I died from AIDS or from a car accident or whatever. I simply knew that I would die consciously, and that created a great celebration in me. With that realization, the significance of ARC took on a very different resonance. It was a doorway to the greatest gift: awareness.

I felt better than I had in years. My body felt and looked great, and I was happier than I had ever allowed myself to be. Because one by one my symptoms had all disappeared and my energy was stronger and more available than it had been in months, my intuition suggested I go for another blood test. It was just a hunch, which came out of nowhere, and my rational mind judged and resisted it. There was no logical possibility that any change could have "miraculously" taken place. I never questioned my future scenario: sooner or later I would develop full-blown AIDS, and a few months after that, I would become a vegetable and die. There was no room for change or choice in that script, because the victim in me, as opposed to the healer, was directing the show. It was an indisputable fact. Just as water boils at one hundred degrees Celsius, Niro will die from AIDS.

But my intuition that this might not be true was reinforced by my friend and counselor Waduda. She has the gift of psychic intuition, and shared with me in session that she felt the disease had left my body. That evening, as I drove back from New York City, I reflected that even though I "knew" Waduda was right, there was still a part of me that did not have the guts to articulate it to anyone. I judged the whole idea as total lunacy, a futile wish that an impossible dream might become a reality. I never questioned the universally accepted belief that AIDS was fatal. How come?

Yet the quiet persistent voice of the healer within faithfully repeated the message: "You are fine, get retested." I heard the message over and over until finally my rational mind gave in, figuring that I had nothing to lose. So I gathered the courage to call, despite a sense that this was going too far, and scheduled a new appointment. Actually, it was not really courage, it was more like boldness.

Driving to the health clinic, I was extremely calm, and had no expectations. I was just responding to the inner voice that had told me I needed to be retested. Yet somewhere in the back of my mind, a small glimmer of hope that I might test negative was present.

Entering the office of my counselor, I knew I was shining. The "poor me" victim was nowhere to be found in that room. My counselor told me later that she was puzzled by my attitude, and

was wondering whether the disease was affecting my brain, or if I
was practicing "wishful thinking."

Throughout the three weeks of waiting for the results (an
improvement over the six-week wait the last time) I did not even
think about the outcome. I was on a sort of high that I can only
describe as a stage of unquestioning trust in "what is so." At one
point my counselor called, which is against protocol because of the
anonymity, and asked if I would come in at once. When I arrived,
she invited me to sit and asked me if I would be willing to be
retested. I responded yes, but wondered why. She explained that
my recent test results came back negative for the HIV antibodies.
She suggested that since the tests showed conflicting results, one of
them must be mistaken and they needed a confirmation of my
present status.

My heart exploded in joy! I knew it. My body had transcended
the disease. I believe it was because I had learned the lesson of my
disease, living from my true essence one moment at a time; therefore the teacher—the disease—could go away.

My counselor drew my blood one more time, to have it retested, and asked me to come back in two weeks. When I returned
for the "official" confirmation that I was indeed HIV-negative, I
immediately made myself available to the medical community. I
knew that I was not special, and that if I could do it, others could
too. I cooperated fully with the doctors, who drew quite a few
pints of blood from me, but unfortunately I never heard from them
again to know what they did with it. I guess I was naïve to have
believed that the medical establishment would be open and willing
to explore the alternative possibilities, which might assist them in
finding a solution to the AIDS crisis. At least I could help them
understand a *part* of healing that might be explored . . . the connection of body, mind, and spirit.

The intuitive part of me accepted the miracle of my healing as
a gift, and I had a strong urge to share what I had learned with
others. The concept seemed so simple. When we are truly committed to live in the present, in acceptance of both ourselves and our
surroundings, miracles can happen. I was so grateful to have re-

ceived the vivid experience of what the enlightened Masters have taught since the beginning of time. I knew intuitively that my healing was an organic result of living in total alignment with the essence of life itself.

My rational mind, on the other hand, was completely baffled. I experienced a numbness similar to what I had felt after I was first diagnosed HIV-positive. It was difficult even to talk about it. I announced it in a shy way to my friends that day at lunch, and then of course I immediately called my children. In a way I was not really amazed, and I didn't really feel lucky either. What I did feel was awkwardness in relating my experience to others, and a deep sense of honor.

My healer within reminded me that an experience like this is not personal. It is a part of the collective experiment of the universe. I was not at liberty to take it for granted and keep it to myself. I was guided to share it, as a way to inspire others faced with a similar challenge and to help change the feeling of doom connected with AIDS. There was no question or hesitation on my part. I knew it was what I needed to do, but in the beginning I had difficulty finding a way to do it. The doctors to whom I had offered my assistance had ignored me, and I was too fragile in the newness of my experience to find a way to express myself with people who were not open to receive me.

At the time I was attached to physical healing, and I realize now that I was quite righteous about it, especially with Nado. Because I was so afraid of losing him, there were times when I acted like I knew all the answers about healing. I was still unaware that one could heal into death; I am grateful to Nado for opening that door for me.

10

Healing
into Death

SEVERAL MONTHS after my healing, on a cold gray November day in 1986, Nado called me and his voice sounded strange. Following a period of separation, we had become friends again. Because we were no longer living together, not trying to play any roles or fulfill any expectations, we were able to rediscover our connection in a brand-new way. "Hi Niro," he said, barely audibly. "Sorry I haven't called you. I've been in Saint Clare's Hospital for the past three weeks. Will you come and visit me?" I was flabbergasted and immediately jumped into my car and drove to New York City.

As I was driving I felt panic mixed with a sense of failure. I prayed to God, making a deal with Her in exchange for Nado's life. "I promise to be good. Please don't let him die." Like a mantra, I repeated it over and over. "Please God, don't let him die. We aren't complete. We still have so much to share together." The love that I felt for him in that moment erased all the bitterness and resentment I had harbored against him. Suddenly all the reasons why we were not together disappeared like the cars passing me on the highway.

When I finally arrived on the AIDS ward of St. Clare's, I was overwhelmed by the feeling of doom that permeated the whole wing. Without being fully conscious of it, I made a vow at that moment to transform the energy surrounding AIDS from one of fear and doom to one of hope and possibility. Nobody deserved to heal in such a dark energy.

As I entered Nado's room, I saw him sitting in a chair with his back toward me. He recognized my footsteps and turned to face me. I was not ready for his ghostly appearance. My heart shattered, and I could hardly breathe. I felt like I had received a tremendous punch in my stomach. Nado looked like he had been in a concentration camp. His huge eyes were staring at me from within his emaciated face. I tried to compose myself and inquire about what had happened, but I was speechless.

As if he could sense my question, Nado began explaining to me that, three weeks earlier, he had collapsed and awakened in this hospital room. He had been diagnosed with *Pneumocystis carinii* pneumonia and toxoplasmosis, both of which were rare diseases common among people with AIDS.

All of my conditioning about how to behave in this kind of situation flew out the window, and the tears just flooded out. I just held him, crying from the depth of my heart. The pain of seeing what had once been a strong, gorgeous, and dynamic man reduced to a shadow of his former self was absolutely unbearable.

After a period of crying together, I felt a huge wave of anger rise inside of me. I was so pissed at that fucking disease which was destroying my beloved. I was unable to hold my emotions in, and I began pacing up and down in that tiny room. I was steaming. Nado watched me silently, and then he smiled, and his smile turned into a laugh. Gently grabbing my hand, he pulled me toward him and held me. Caressing my face like he so often had before, he told me how precious and refreshing my honesty was. He had felt so isolated by the denial from the majority of the people around him. He felt alienated from his friends and their strained attempts at encouragement and comfort as a way to avoid their own fear and discomfort concerning death.

I began visiting him every other day. In the beginning I was constantly advising him what to do, what not to do, practically what to think. He patiently accepted it, knowing that it was my way of loving him. I wanted so badly for him to get well. Because they had to hook him up with tubes to take care of his bodily functions, the scene was becoming more horrifying every day. I watched the two parts of me, each experiencing the situation so differently. On one side was my present adult, and the healer within, calmly accepting what was happening, and responding creatively. On the other side was my inner child, with her many survival masks, doing whatever she could to avoid that sense of helplessness that would overwhelm me every time I entered Nado's room.

As Nado's body became sicker, he became more and more obsessed with getting out of the hospital. Even though he was receiving the right medication and the appropriate care, the energy of the hospital was so foreign and in such total opposition to his spiritual beliefs, and his genuine vital needs, that it was literally killing him. "If I stay here," he warned me, "I'm gonna die soon, and this is not where I want to die."

Nado had a dream of returning to his birthplace in Holland for his father's seventieth birthday. A celebration was scheduled for the end of November, and his entire family would be there. He had been planning the trip for months prior to his hospitalization as a way to complete many issues with his father, and that was an opportunity he did not want to miss.

Unfortunately, he was still too sick to be released from the hospital immediately, because his fever was too high. In order for him to be released, the fever needed to be below one hundred degrees Fahrenheit. So we started to focus on specific meditation and visualization techniques to bring his body temperature down.

In the meantime we chose a deadline to motivate us, and I made airline reservations for the both of us since I had decided that I would fly back to Europe with him. Nado was very moved when he discovered my intention to fly with him, and it created an opening for him to tell me how he finally understood what I had meant about merging. He shared how in a strange way it was happening between us. Because nothing was in the way of our connection, we were both nourished by it. It wasn't about making plans for the future, or dwelling in the past, but drinking in the preciousness of each moment we had together. We knew that we had very few moments left together, and so we stopped postponing fully expressing the love we had for each other.

The first three days of meditation and visualization were

magic. Nado's body responded right away. His healing was also supported by various herbs sent to him from a healer in California. Then suddenly all of his symptoms worsened severely. Just after returning home from a visit to him, I received a phone call from the hospital to come at once. The hospital personnel were very concerned about the decline in his health, and feared that Nado might not make it through the night.

When I arrived at the hospital, he was barely breathing; each breath seemed to demand such extreme effort. When I saw him, I freaked out. I asked the nurse what could be done, and the answer was that they had done everything they could, and we just had to wait. So I tried. I sat near the bed and held Nado's hand, focusing on giving him all the force and light that I could. I visualized a clear channel of light pouring from my heart into each of his cells. I became very warm, and I felt such a strong energy coming through me that I could not stay still. Trusting what was happening, I instinctively began to rub his legs, which were strangely cold, even though he had a high fever. I massaged his right arm, but was unable to massage both, because the left one was covered with shingles. I was no longer identifying with the painful emotions of seeing his body so afflicted. I was just doing what needed to be done. I massaged every part of his body that I possibly could, revitalizing it with aliveness, and recharging it with love. It was so obvious how much his body needed those loving strokes.

I did all I could to shower my beloved with unconditional love, and then I waited. My energy was spent. Around five o'clock in the morning he opened his eyes and smiled at me. He softly asked what time it was and if we were leaving soon, as planned. I began to laugh and laugh, unable to answer, and he just watched me, not really understanding my outburst of energy. Then he started laughing too, and life force came back into his eyes. The shadows began disappearing from his emaciated face, and his exquisite beauty was still so apparent, yet with no masks hiding any of it. I went and lay next to him, and we fell asleep together holding each other tightly. Little did I know that it would be the last time we would hold each other in that way.

The next day, we talked and talked like never before. He shared his memories of his childhood, and his journey from Indonesia where he grew up to Holland and eventually to America. He shared his shame about his bisexuality, and his guilt for having infected me with the virus. He told me that he finally understood what I meant when I spoke about letting go into love. I remember so precisely what he said. "Niro, you have opened the door to my heart. It was closed so tight for such a long time, and now that it has cracked open, it will never close again." That was all I needed to hear. My heart was totally open as well. Nothing else was needed. In that moment everything was complete.

For the next two days I packed, preparing for our journey. We spoke several times a day, taking care of all the details. Nado's fever finally broke and his temperature was stabilizing at around ninety-nine degrees Fahrenheit.

In order for Nado to be released, he needed to walk out of the building on his own. I was so moved by his valiant effort as he hobbled with his cane down the long corridor. He did not allow us to hold him or help him. He was on his own. All I could do was send him all of my emotional support. Slowly and steadily he wobbled closer and closer to the doorway. When he finally crossed the threshold into the freedom of the outside world, my friend Vasant caught him in his arms and lovingly helped him into the front seat of the car.

The staff at the airport was so supportive. They gave us a whole row of seats, so that Nado could lie down; I sat on the aisle one row in front of him. During the flight, Nado began to experience some delirium. He started rambling, sometimes quite loudly, and his fever shot right up. I was afraid that the trip might have been too much for Nado's weak constitution, and that he would die right there in the airplane, thousands of miles from any kind of medical support. I felt more helpless than ever.

We finally landed in Brussels, where a wheelchair was ready and waiting. I placed his hat on his head and draped his scarf around his neck to hide the Kaposi's sarcoma lesion on the side of his face. I knew he did not want to frighten his family, and as usual he wanted to look his best, which he did. As I silently pushed him in his wheelchair, he had the air of a king on his throne.

We crossed the doors after passing through customs, and his family was waiting there expectantly. Their faces reflected the shock and concern they felt at seeing their loved one looking extremely sick, with his large eyes ravishing in his shrunken face. I returned to collect the baggage as Nado was absorbed by all those "foreign" people speaking Dutch, and suddenly I felt like a complete stranger.

A short while later, his brother parked his car in front of the exit and carried his baggage to it. Nado looked so happy, speaking his native language, surrounded by his family, but I felt awkward, and separate. I didn't know how to act or what to do with myself. When it was time for us to say good-bye, we both felt very weird embracing; since he was sitting, I had to bend down to kiss his cheek.

Because he wanted to assure his family of his well-being, he refused assistance and walked out of the airport on his own. Using his cane, he wobbled so much as he took each step that I was afraid he would fall. Finally the automatic doors opened and, without looking back, he passed through the doorway and into his brother's car. That is the way Nado walked out of my life.

Several weeks later, at two in the morning, Nado's brother called to inform me that Nado had died peacefully in his sleep. The following day his body was cremated as he had requested. His brother told me that Nado had asked that my photograph be placed on his heart, next to one of our beloved master Osho. Nado died in February 1987—at the age of forty-two, just as he had predicted.

Today I feel Nado vibrantly present as an important part of my life, but in a brand-new way. The gift of not being with him at the moment of his death was that it kept his presence alive and real for me. In a way, I never fully accepted the fact that he was gone. There was a part of me that still believed Nado was living somewhere in Europe, that hoped that one day we would be reunited.

Writing these pages has given me the opportunity to finally let go of the dream and close that chapter of my life. It is the past, and it no longer exists. What remains in the present is a deep sense of gratitude for our journey together, and the gift that my connection with Nado was in my life.

11

Sharing
a New Purpose

BECAUSE THE NEGATIVE NEWS surrounding AIDS was still making the headlines, I knew that it was urgent to go public with my story as soon as possible. I had to keep my promise. The first step was to create a ten-week course especially designed for people with AIDS, ARC, or HIV infection. The concept was very simple. The group was open to ten participants; it would meet once a week for three hours, to meditate, explore self-discovery processes, and share the healing journey. Once a week each participant would see me for a private therapy session, to integrate the group work and to explore a more personal psychological aspect of the journey. I designed the course this way because I value the personal work in private session as well as the nourishment that is available in a group. I did not base the ten-week course on any traditional therapeutic approach, but rather on acceptance, recognition, respect, and love, which I believe is the best healing remedy there is.

I was invited to speak at a small PWA support group in Manhattan, and the reaction of the men who were there was extremely beautiful. Several of them called me the next day to thank me for the ray of hope and light that I had brought into their lives. They were so grateful to be able finally to verify what they had intuitively known inside, namely that AIDS is not one-hundred-percent fatal, as the media and the medical community would have us believe. I felt as if my entire life had been a preparation for sharing my experience with people who were ready to be inspired and assisting them in integrating healing into their own life.

Because the program I was developing still did not have a name, one of my clients with AIDS came up with a name for it. I had told him that I wanted a title that included self-healing and AIDS. That night he fell asleep and in a semi-dream state he conceived the name Self Healing AIDS-Related Experience, with the acronym S.H.A.R.E. It resonated strongly with me. The only alteration I made was changing the word experience to experiment, because that was what it truly was. We then incorporated as a not-for-profit organization under the official title The Foundation for the Self Healing AIDS-Related Experiment.

The first ten-week course started in September 1987 with five participants who were HIV-positive. As of this writing, three are still asymptomatic and are serving the AIDS community through volunteer work. From there the next ten-week programs organically grew, and I was feeling happier than I had in my entire life. But as is my tendency, I overextended myself and let the demands of my schedule grow out of hand, into a level of insanity. Part of my work was visiting patients in the hospital, and I found it extremely difficult to say no to someone in that situation. As part of the program, I wanted to create a very close and intimate relationship with each of the participants; as a result I lived, slept, and even dreamt S.H.A.R.E. Once again, I had to learn a new set of boundaries, yet it was difficult since the epidemic was creating such a level of urgency.

In order to nurture myself and stay centered, I participated in workshops with my dear friend and teacher Amitabh. I was so impressed by the way Amitabh worked with people, assisting them to move through their fear and take their next step, that I invited him to come and work with the participants of the ten-week course. He accepted enthusiastically and immediately conceived the title "Who Heals" for the new workshop we were designing together. The foundation continued to grow, and we expanded to the West Coast.

There were many days when I had discouragement and doubts, and was totally overwhelmed by the dimensions of the job, but my inner voice of integrity kept showing me the way. After three years of facilitating workshops throughout the United States and Europe, it is becoming clearer to me that what I am creating is a safe place for people to reconnect with their own spirituality and spiritual family. I do not mean "spiritual" in the sense of religion, or dogma, but more in terms of the natural urge of the soul to experience and overflow with love. To me, that is the essence of healing.

Today, the vision dearest to my heart is the creation of a residential healing and meditation center. This would be a place where we can choose to live and die consciously, based on what we know in our hearts. I have founded the Healing Home in East Hampton, New York, as the first step to realizing this vision.

Since my healing, I have had the privilege of sharing my experience with hundreds of people around the world. I have no words to describe the inspiration, love, and respect that I have received as a result. I will always be grateful for the beauty, the recognition, and the light that shines in each one of our meetings. It guides us to keep going on the journey . . . despite our minds.

2

LESSONS FROM
A JOURNEY

12

Our Wake-up Call

*Rejoice at your inner powers for they are
the makers of wholeness and holiness in
you.*

—HIPPOCRATES

WHEN LIFE presents us with the challenge of a life-threatening illness, our instinct tells us to heal. It is common sense. Why then has tapping into our healing energy become so difficult for us?

Because most of us are not in tune with ourselves and our bodies, our ability to listen to the message sent by our physical body has become distorted. As we have become more "civilized" and moved farther and farther away from the natural flow of life, our healing powers have faded away as the result of neglect. We rely more and more on the "magical" symptom suppressors of modern medicine. For centuries we have given away our healing powers to the sorcerer, the medicine woman, the doctor. We fell asleep and lost our ability to listen to our bodies, totally unaware that we would become disconnected from our responsibility for the disharmony between our physical, emotional, and spiritual selves.

When we are physically suffering, we usually want the disease to go away as quickly as possible, and are ready to undergo the most extreme treatments in an effort to get rid of the symptoms. In our society we have denied the power of accepting the sometimes painful message of the physical body, which motivates us to change. By treating the symptoms exclusively, we are only masking the problem which is the source of the symptoms.

A client recently told me that he feels he finally understands the core of what I am teaching. To put it roughly in his words, the healing process is not about seeking results; rather it is about living life to the fullest, and healing those issues which are the source of the illness. He told how he had misused his precious energy worrying and focusing on curing the symptoms, and that it had only intensified them. By working with his core issues of guilt and shame, and by letting go of his attachment to results, he had now begun to value his life simply as it was. By accepting the painful moments, and allowing the energy to be released, he was able to keep the pain from becoming chronic.

Sharing the details of my personal healing experience with someone is easy. Yet if someone really wants to receive the essence of my experience, it requires a great willingness on their part. What I usually encounter is curiosity, but rarely total commitment. Why is that? In each person the desire to get rid of the disease is genuine. They say they will do anything to heal, but when I invite them to practice a specific daily technique, they lose interest after a short time. When they begin to examine their lives to discover the source of their illness, and it becomes too uncomfortable, they find any excuse to stop. I have even encountered people who are aware of the source of their disease, but still would rather subject their body to symptom-suppressing poison than change the attitude or behavior which is a co-factor of the disease itself.

Dr. Bernie Siegel, a well-known surgeon and best-selling author, noted in his book *Love, Medicine and Miracles* that the majority of cancer patients would rather undergo a serious operation under total anesthesia than take charge of their life. They would rather "go under the knife" than change their diet, give up their addictions, and exercise more.

Why is it that even though someone knows what needs to be healed in his life, and his intuition is guiding him to take specific steps on his healing journey, he spends his energy justifying why he is not doing it?

The reason is fear. Fear of pain and fear of dying. When we postpone facing our fear and discomfort we miss another opportunity to take charge of our lives. The mind is like a Ping-Pong ball, bouncing between the two opposing beliefs about our condition, and creating havoc within us.

ONE: The situation is uncomfortable, and very soon it may become painful. I need to take action in order to avoid the pain.

TWO: If we change our attitude or behavior it will feel strange and uncomfortable. It may be scary, too, because we are not used to it.

ONE: Oh-oh. Pain and discomfort again. Maybe we can postpone a little longer.

We use our creativity in an escapist way. Our bodies send us the signals, but we do not listen to them in the early stages when they are mild. We ignore the message and keep pushing our bodies, judging our need for rest and rejuvenation as weakness. We keep pushing, keep working, keep partying, until eventually we force our bodies into serious illness.

When Julian became aware of his HIV status, he was a heavy smoker and a pot addict. He was dieting, meditating, reading all the self-help books, and making great efforts to take care of himself. But he would not stop smoking tobacco or pot, as if he were totally oblivious to the impact of those habits on someone with a fragile immune system. Even though he was doing more and more exercise, meditation, and self-treatment, he felt the opposite of what he was expecting; he experienced more anger, resentment, and misery. It brought him closer to the point where he had to face the action he was *not* taking, and the cost he paid for it in his life and well-being.

I invited him to quit smoking, not by sheer will power, but by going totally *into* smoking, with full awareness, and observing exactly what he was feeling when he was doing it. First he discovered how difficult it was for him to be fully aware in this way; then he realized that he really did not like the taste of tobacco or pot, or the effect they had on him, but that his behavior was just a habit based on the memory of how good and relaxed smoking used to make him feel. However, those feelings were no longer available.

Then he realized how unnecessary it was to keep on doing something he did not enjoy, just because he was used to it. He felt he had turned into a machine over which he had no control. Regaining that control was hard work, because he then had to face the emotions that he had always tried to avoid by smoking—mainly anger and sadness. But the new experience of cleansing and the sense of being in charge of his life finally gave him the strength to make that passage. After having tried many treatments over more than twelve years, Julian quit smoking in less than three weeks.

Another fear which is a major source of illness is the fear of living, and the unconscious desire to die. I see many of my clients achieving honesty with themselves and finally embracing the fact that they don't want a life that seems pointless and without challenge. Because they are afraid to change, however, their new awareness gets lost in an array of justifications and rationalizations about why they are not healing.

A life-threatening challenge is our inescapable opportunity to look at our undeniable mortality. It is an open door to a totally new way of experiencing life moment by moment. That challenge instantly leads us to the next level of consciousness available. Although disease seems destructive on the physical level, it offers an opportunity to let go of everything that is false in us. When we allow ourselves to say yes to our real feelings, the disease can be released, and we can heal into life or death. The lesson has been understood.

We may not have control over the evolution of a disease in our body, but we do have a choice to change the quality of our life and to create a difference in how we deal with the physical symptoms. When I was diagnosed I understood in a flash that my life had changed totally. I was pressured by time, by a *dead*line, and I did not postpone. I finally did what I needed to do:

- Put myself on the top of the list
- Live in the now
- Live totally
- Live in gratitude
- Let go of the subtle yet paralyzing guilt and self-denial that were in the way of allowing peace and harmony within me

It may have been simple, but it certainly was not easy. I know in my heart that, because I changed my attitude toward life, I experienced a healing of my entire being, which resulted in my physical body healing as well. Again, once the lesson is learned, the teacher has completed its purpose and can move on.

Those of you who interpret my healing as something I did—as in "Niro *healed herself* of ARC"—will be missing what I have to share with you. It was not something *I did*. It was an allowing, a surrender into the reality of my mortality, and then the doing was a change of the quality of my life from that new awareness. *The physical healing was a bonus.* My healing was the result of a letting go, not the result of controlling my physical body.

Remember that healing is not a doing, it is an allowing. It is the open door to a different dimension of life. The key to this door is pain. It is an opportunity to meet the part of ourselves that we did not know existed. Healing is an opening to meditation. The disease is the tool that keeps us awake, and on our path toward our maximum potential. It is an opportunity to become what Bernie Siegel calls an "exceptional patient." They are individuals who use their diagnosis as a springboard into a totally new way of life. Life becomes a celebration of each moment as a gift, and is no longer perceived as the enemy. Healing is a journey through inner storms of confusion and doubt on the way to inner silence. It is in this silence that we meet the healer within, and receive the wisdom of our heart.

My healing journey was one of honesty with myself. Through it I discovered a new form of freedom by dropping all pretense— including the pretense of not having pretenses. It has been an exquisite and painful communion with myself. I finally looked at all those parts of me that I had judged as unacceptable and embraced them as pieces of who I am. I said yes to the dance between the magnificent, capable, and divine being that I am and the hopeless, fearful, and controlling survivor that I am as well.

In this section of the book I will share with you the lessons I received from my journey, as a way for you to discover what is available to you on your journey. My invitation to you is to take what resonates for you as truth, and leave the rest. Do not try to go against your own *truth* in order to get results. The results will evolve through your own self-empowerment, when you trust what resonates in you.

We will explore our "no" to all our hidden emotions like anger, despair, and fear, including our terror of physical pain. We will examine our inability to express our real needs or feelings, as a way to make ourselves available to our "yes," and the wisdom of our inner voice.

We will explore our tendency to perceive our universe as a realm of extreme polarities, as a world of either/or, and discover that a place in between exists. For example, some people look at a glass of water and see it as half full, while others see it as half empty. I see it as simultaneously half full *and* half empty. Seeing both is being aware of the whole, going beyond the either/or concept. It is in this state of wholeness that healing is available to us. In this state we can remember who we truly are, accepting the good with the bad and recognizing that we know more about our healing than any therapist, doctor, or specialist.

Remember to choose a journal as one of your healing tools and to keep it in a safe place but one that is easily accessible. Your journal will serve two purposes. The first is to record your thoughts, feelings, dreams, and anything else of importance in the day-to-day progression of your journey. Keep your journal with you, especially at work, where so often we get overstressed, and our fears get reactivated. Use the journal as a silent partner that can receive all of your feelings of anger, frustration, and sadness, as a way to release those negative emotions.

The second purpose of your journal will be to serve as a

passive partner in the self-discovery process described in these pages. Some of the processes are extremely simple, consisting of making lists of all the choices or "ingredients" you have available to you. Once you have them written in front of you in black and white, instead of floating around in your head, they become clearer and simpler. You will also be encouraged to create a "prescription" for your healing, and design your own daily awareness routine.

Use your creativity to decorate the cover of your journal and make it your own. Make it personal and unique. Remember, your journal is sacred and private. Please do not show the contents of your journal to anyone. It has a very special energy. It is not appropriate to share it with anyone else, until that day when you feel confident enough to fully reveal yourself.

Healing is a very private journey, especially in the beginning. This is when the most drastic change of behavior is necessary, and it is often threatening to the people in our lives. It is sometimes difficult to see that, even though they love us, they have plenty of preconceptions about what we should and should not do, and how we should be. They may be threatened by our new attitudes and try to control us with well-meaning advice. Share your healing journey only with those people who are on the same path, and can understand your process—for example, people with whom you feel aligned in healing circles, twelve-step meetings, and support groups.

Your journal will become a concrete reflection of the rapid growth that will certainly take place the moment you commit yourself to your healing journey. If you have not done so yet, I invite you to stop for a moment, close your eyes, and make a commitment with yourself to participate fully in these processes, which are designed to access the healer within.

Healing is discovering who we are in each moment, and saying yes to it, without trying to change anything. Change happens on its own anyway, if we simply let it be. Healing takes the courage to let go of the decisions we made when we were discovering behaviors around us and learning them as well—these decisions come from our need to survive, and to open the door to the question of the unknown. By emptying ourselves of repressed emotion, old conditioning, and limited thoughts, we become available to the guidance of the healer within. My invitation to you is to open yourself to receive the message of your wake-up call, and to start living it today.

13

Energy

When energy flows, overflows, without any motivation, it becomes delight. That is the moment when you have started pouring into God. And the moment you start to pour into God, God starts pouring into you. It happens simultaneously.

—WILLIAM BLAKE

IN THIS UNIVERSE we live in, everything is energy. Some energy is very dense and solid—like our physical body, or a tree, or a rock. Other energy is a little less dense and comes in the liquid form, like the ocean, the rain, or the blood in our veins. Then there is a finer, less dense vibration of energy in the gaseous state, which can be visible like clouds or smoke, or invisible, like oxygen, nitrogen, and all the other invisible gases.

Energy is partially defined in the dictionary as having the force to take action; the strength and power used to produce a result. On one level it is simply that. When we are tired we often say "I don't have the energy" to accomplish a task. Or before attempting a strenuous challenge, we think "I better preserve my energy." Einstein expanded the definition through his understanding that all matter is energy. Even a rock is pulsating energy responding to that universal cycle of contraction and expansion.

We can easily recognize most forms of energy in the physical dimension, yet we are constantly reacting and responding to more ethereal forms of energy. We can feel this energy even if it is not physically concrete. Emotions are an example of ethereal energy

which creates reactions in us. For instance, we know when someone around is contracted or expanded, angry or pleased, without
them saying a word. Everywhere nowadays we hear people speaking about energy. Healing energy, love energy, psychic energy, positive and negative energy. Certain concepts and terminology I will
be using may be new for some of you, so I will attempt to be as
clear as possible, yet I will only be reminding you of what you
already know on another "energy level."

Connecting with Our Energy

Try this exercise for a conscious experience of your own pulsating
energy. Shake one of your hands for one minute, as strong and fast
as you can, and then after the minute has passed, abruptly stop and
tune into the way your hand feels. Go ahead and try it.

How does it feel? It probably feels much bigger and very alive.
Now imagine what it would feel like if you did the same with your
entire body. If you are willing to vigorously shake your body for
fifteen minutes with your eyes closed, you will have an experience
of your physical energy in its full expansion. This exercise is actually the first stage of the Kundalini meditation, designed by Osho
for the modern Western Man, that I teach in my workshops. Kundalini energy means life-force energy, and throughout the ages
many masters have designed various yogic and meditation techniques for us to get in touch with it. When we are in touch with our
life force, it is exhilarating because we recognize that we are much
more powerful than our disease.

As part of understanding the way energy works, let's take as a
hypothesis for now that energy moves in a circular pattern, either
vertically or horizontally. We can see it everywhere around us in
the physical world. In the life of a tree, for instance: a seed is
planted, it grows, becomes a tree, and blossoms, then the seeds fall
from the tree and return to the earth. It is the cycle of life and
death.

Damming Our Energy

Human beings are strange animals because we believe we can control the circle of energy directed to and from us. When we try to control energy, it is distorted. For instance, when positive or negative energy has been directed at us, it will affect us positively or negatively and simply move on. That is the nature of energy. But our attempts to control it can make the energy harmful to us, because we tense our bodies and hold the energy in. When we are tense, we are always on the defensive, ready for the worst. Healing requires that the body and mind be relaxed. If we simply allow the energy that is directed at us to pass through us, not resisting or controlling it, it will not affect us as strongly, regardless of whether it is positive or negative.

When we let go of control, we become a channel for the current of energy, which then is like a river constantly flowing through us. When we control or repress the flow of energy, we create a dam, and the river of energy becomes a stagnant swamp. This repressed energy will build inside of us and continue to try to find a way out. If the healthy channels have been denied, it may eventually come out through the skin via a rash, or shingles, or a cancerous tumor for example.

When Sally started my ten-week course, she was in a wheelchair, or sometimes walking with crutches. At the last session in East Hampton, she was jumping above the waves.

In a support group two years later, I noticed that, even though she was extremely moved by what was happening in the room and in herself, she was sitting in a tight position and her jaw was clenched. I could see that she was once again in great physical pain and that walking was a great effort for her.

When I asked her how she was doing, she replied in a complaining tone that the emotions were wearing her out. I simply reminded her that maybe it was the opposite; maybe it was *controlling* her emotions that exhausted her. She laughed and said, "I forgot again." She transformed in front of our eyes, and in less than five minutes all the pain in her legs was gone—she had released the energy that was stuck there. It is so important to remember that it sometimes takes several reminders to create a new behavior.

Healing is the pure flow of light energy. It is the harmonious balance of energy, beyond control and judgment, beyond what we like and dislike. Healing energy makes us feel that all our senses are awake, that our awareness is heightened. As our energy vibrates powerfully through us, there is no end and no beginning. It is always available. This state of harmonious balance is what we are here to learn and experience at this state of evolution.

Creative Energy of the Soul

When our energy is balanced it is creative. When it is unbalanced, it is reactive. Reactive energy is our mind's response to the conditioning of the past. Creative energy happens when we are focused on what is happening now. When we align ourselves with our creative energy, we align ourselves with the energy of the soul.

The soul is timeless, as opposed to the mind, which is limited by time. It is in the energy of the soul that we all are one. In this energy our individual identities disappear and our uniqueness arises. This is where we merge, and where we accept what is so. It is in this energy that we heal and, as if by magic, our physical body responds.

To understand this process it is helpful to first understand the creative process. Physical life begins as a thought, a mental image or idea. This thought becomes the creative impetus for physical creation. It is then empowered by an emotional attitude which motivates the idea into action. It is this action which carries the thought into the reality of the physical realm.

A wonderful metaphor for this creative process is symbolized in the arts. An artist or musician is divinely inspired by an idea, which seemingly comes from nowhere or what they sometimes call "the ethers." He or she then filters the idea through their personal passion, which motivates them to manifest the inspiration on the physical plane. Hours and hours of hard work result in the creation of an exquisitely beautiful painting or musical composition. The artist has literally channeled beauty from the ethereal realms of the heavens to the physical dimension of the earth.

Scientists and inventors act in much the same way, often working exclusively on a hunch, or an intuitive impulse. As our collective consciousness expands, we learn how to understand and use energy as a tool of progress. The scientific accomplishments throughout the last century alone are astronomical. Tools of communication, which send our voices and images across the planet via satellite, are helping to unite the world. Exploration into outer space, and into inner space, is helping us understand who we are as beings and how we fit into the bigger picture. As we continue to learn how to master energy via atomic energy, high technology, computers, and lasers, we must bear in mind that they can be used to kill or to heal. The choice is up to us.

Distorted Energy and Disease

Disease follows the same formula of physical manifestation. It begins as a thought, separating it from the wholeness of spirit. This thought is then fed by the "negative" emotions such as fear, resentment, guilt, and greed, which empower the disease to manifest. Emotions which are repressed have an even greater effect on the physical body, because the energy gets stuck and the life force is unable to flow in its natural cycle of contraction and expansion. When physical symptoms appear, they are not the first signs of disease, as some may believe; in actuality they are the last warning signs of a process that began much earlier.

We have disease because our bodies work perfectly well. When we are diseased, our bodies are simply responding to the distorted thoughts and decisions that we hold or repress in our minds. We usually judge that our bodies are not functioning well when we are sick, but we rarely look at the source: the neglect, abuse, and general maltreatment we subject them to.

Health is a natural state of being. It flourishes when our energy is flowing in its natural harmonious balance. This is why, when we are faced with a physical disease, it is vital to release the repressed emotions and return to the source, to the thought or decision which "inspired" the physical manifestation of the disease. Decisions like "I am not worthy" or "Life is a struggle" can set the tone for our lives. Deeply embedded guilt about our sexuality, for example, can lead to the pattern of acting out and punishment, which can manifest itself physically as a sexually transmitted disease, such as herpes or AIDS.

Scientists and doctors are finally beginning to recognize the importance of the mind-body connection in terms of healing and disease, as in the science of psychoimmunology, which Dr. Joan Borysenko has written about in her book *Minding the Body, Mending the Mind*. Denial of the connection between our physical body and our thoughts and emotions has created the monstrous medical industry, with its high-priced hospitals, practitioners, and drugs. The appearance of so many "incurable" diseases such as cancer and AIDS is contributing to changing the medical monopoly. Some patients are now being encouraged by their caregivers to use positive imagery, laughter, and life-affirming attitudes as tools in the healing process. These techniques of balancing the emotions can be of great benefit in turning the tide of disease.

Emotional Energy

Emotion is simply energy vibrating at different frequencies. We can describe it as E-motion: energy in motion. Anger vibrates at one level, sadness at another, joy at another. The moment we are aware of this, we can realign our inner harmony through meditation and very specific exercises, designed to work with the emotional body. We then can determine which kind of energy contributes to our well-being, and which kind is destructive.

For instance, remember a time when someone, perhaps an authority figure, reproached you for doing something wrong, and he or she had a lot of anger toward you? Remember your specific emotional reaction to that energy of anger? Now imagine a gentle, loving teacher explaining to you with kindness and patience that you have made a mistake, and lovingly giving you feedback on how to avoid that mistake in the future. Notice what response you have to that energy. Those are the different energy vibrations. That is why some people say that a person has "good vibes" or "bad vibes." What they are really saying is, "The way I feel when I am around that person is good" or "bad."

For centuries, we have repressed our emotional energy, permitting only the "positive" ones like love, hope, and courage to be celebrated. We have disowned the "negative" emotions, like anger, sadness, and fear. As a result, we have created a world of control, separation, and enmity, far from the harmony and oneness that is available to us in our merging experiences.

Energy as Life Force

Energy is the miracle of being alive, right now, this second, and we can use that energy in any direction we like. We can direct it into anger, or we can channel it into love. It is the same energy; we can use it however we like. It is our choice. When we use our energy to resist, our entire life falls into a pattern of resistance, and our energy does not flow. Because the energy is contained, it eventually forms a stagnant, rotting swamp. Again, we choose this unhappy state, usually unconsciously; no one is doing it to us. The way we control our energy is by saying no to life. When we are willing to say yes, our energy can be free, and in order to say yes we need to wake up.

We have been conditioned to use our energy for resistance, defense, and separation. This is supported by an endless series of standards coming from our childhood programming about right or wrong. Once we have absorbed this programming as our own, we rarely question it, and we accept it as our "truth." It is not until we are faced with some kind of life crisis that we begin to ask what parts of our programming are valuable in our lives, and what parts no longer serve us.

Energy is life force. It needs to be respected as a very unique and sacred gift. Unfortunately, it is not something that we are taught in school. I disrespected life force and wasted so much precious energy, so many times, by saying no to what life was offering me. Those memories are very painful to me, but in a strange way, I will never forget them, because they served as powerful lessons.

We have very skillfully used our energy in a limited and destructive way for centuries. Now the signs are all around us, and we have seen the writing on the wall. We have gone too far, nearly past the point of no return. It is time to change direction, to say yes and to use our energy in an expansive way, the way of the heart.

14

The Dance of
Contraction and Expansion

*Verily you are suspended like scales be-
tween your sorrow and your joy. Only
when you are empty, are you at a standstill
and balanced.*

—KAHLIL GIBRAN,
The Prophet

AS I LEARNED by observing the ocean, all energy is governed by
the universal law of contraction and expansion. Night and day,
winter and summer, birth and death, positive and negative, masculine and feminine. This natural balance of opposites, referred to
as yin and yang in the Chinese Tao, rules everything in this dual-
istic universe of ours. We only have to observe the ebb and flow of
the ocean tide to appreciate the beauty and perfection of that dance
in nature.

As humans we have distorted the dance. We have unexpressed
judgments and attachments to expansion. We prefer vacation over
work, and we value our rest sometimes more than our full creativity. We often choose security over living fully and exploring new
possibilities. We have stopped accepting the natural flow of contraction and expansion, and have tried foolishly to control it, because we fear that contraction is something bad. Ironically, that
fear itself begets more contraction, and so we become more and
more dependent on artificial sources of expansion.

Contraction and expansion are the two ingredients of the

whole, and we have lost our acceptance of what is whole. When we wake up to that awareness, we can then relax into letting go of the illusion that we have the ability to control it, and live in the natural flow.

As embryos in our mother's womb, we respond naturally to the harmonious dance between the opposite energies. Then comes the trauma of birth, upsetting the perfect rhythm and creating the first unnatural contraction. As babies we are still greatly influenced by the natural pulse of life, as we play and nap, eat and defecate, laugh and cry. It isn't until Mommy and Daddy begin to train us that we start to lose touch with our natural rhythm. In order to continue to earn our parents' love and "fit in," we quickly learn to behave like good little girls and boys. We learn that if we cry our parents respond by bringing us food or cuddling us, and that if we urinate or defecate on the floor or in the crib it displeases them. We learn to adapt to the circumstances of our environment by controlling our bodily functions as conditioned responses to our parents' cue.

The reason we adapt ourselves is simply to survive. We try our best to become the person our parents, our teachers, and our priests want us to be. We end up as a tense series of knots, perceiving life through filters of learned behavior. We get lost in the labyrinth of being "good" and feeling unworthy. We are no longer human *beings,* but human *doings.* Our natural rhythm is broken. In this imbalanced state, we repress our natural energy, our joy, love, anguish, and fear. We are no longer able to simply express what is so for us in the present moment.

In order for life to dance its dance, there needs to be space for our natural rhythm. Because most of us have fallen out of sync with that natural rhythm, we falsely believe that we can control it. When we are in contraction we will do almost anything to find expansion, in an effort to feel "good."

When we are babies, sucking our mother's nipple or a bottle can bring us that sense of love and security. Our mother's touch, or our father's embrace can establish that sense of peace and expansion. As we grow up, however, these experiences are quickly replaced with surrogate sources of the sense of expansion, often quite distorted. Food, alcohol, recreational drugs, sex, TV, shopping, any kind of "recreation" can be used to re-create that sense of expansion. But these temporary "highs" cannot counterbalance the deep low in the core of our being, the contraction we try desperately to escape from. This contraction offers us the opportunity to look within, yet most of us are afraid and run from it. It is my experience that this compulsion to live exclusively in expansion is one of the major causes of addiction in our severely addicted society.

Recreation and Addiction

Some of us use recreational drugs and alcohol, others use sex with people we don't love. Some of us may buy designer clothes, drive a fast car, or take out a bigger mortgage on a more expensive house. Some of us, like myself, indulge in chocolate and sweets, others spend hours watching TV and movies or playing games and national pastimes. Many of us dedicate our entire life to working at a job we hate just to earn the money to pay for these recreations. We work fifty weeks a year to pay for the mortgage, the possessions, the status symbols, and then take costly vacations in an effort to relax and forget. We will use any form of recreation, which is literally a re-creating of the sensation of expansion, to escape feeling our package of suppressed emotion, including shame, anger, fear, and sadness.

Most of us spend our energy seeking the highs in an effort to avoid the lows. Unfortunately, these false highs are not really nourishing, since they are generated by external sources with the intention of helping us escape ourselves. True expansion originates from within us and flows outward as an expression of who we are.

I'm not saying that we should not enjoy recreation. For me a delectable cup of vanilla Swiss almond ice cream, a delicious swim in the ocean, or a romantic dinner by candlelight can certainly be considered a true source of expansion, as long as it is not used as an obsessive way of avoiding my feelings.

Expansion comes from being, not doing. When we are busy doing, we miss the natural expansion of being. Often, once we've finished doing whatever it is we do to feel good, we crave the experience again and again because we are never really satisfied. For me, I desire more chocolate; for someone else it may be another drink, a faster car, or a bigger house. Sometimes we may feel even more contracted than we did before we experienced our false high—when we are hungover, for instance, or in debt from a shopping spree, or lying in bed feeling even more separate and alone after our sex partner leaves. This pattern creates and sustains addiction, a problem of epidemic proportion in our culture today.

Addiction is our mind's attachment to a particular substance or behavior in the belief that it is going to create the sense of expansion that we crave. Drugs give the user an initial glimpse at bliss, but this cannot be sustained artificially. Alcohol relaxes people so that they can temporarily drop their fears and inhibitions and experience a feeling of freedom and expansion. Users of alcohol may allow their repressed feelings or behaviors to surface in public, only to judge themselves harshly for this in the daylight of sobriety. The consequent sense of contraction from this self-judgment and shame creates the need for more alcohol as a way to escape the contraction; this leads to a vicious cycle of artificial contraction and expansion.

This should not be confused with the natural cycle of contraction and expansion, which creates a sense of harmony and balance in our lives. This natural cycle is self-healing. The artificial or controlled cycle brings chaos and adds to one's sense of confusion and despair. It is self-destructive.

Sexual Addiction

Another addiction which is far more rampant than is currently acknowledged in our society is sexual addiction. Like intravenous drug addiction, this problem is directly connected to the spread of AIDS as a disease. Like other addictions, it is the result of the search for artificial expansion as a way to avoid contraction, yet it is tricky because its behavior patterns have often been confused with the actions of love.

Our culture has presented sex in romantic fashion masquerading as love, but sex and love are two distinct energies. Love is natural expansion. Sex, when it is used simply as a "fix," is an artificial expansion. Unlike love, which comes from an intimacy with ourselves and our partners, sex without love or respect comes from the conditioning of our mind. It comes from the past and has very little to do with the present moment or the partner we are with. As a way of avoiding the vulnerability of intimacy, we project our mind's fantasies onto the partner with whom we are acting out our sexual or relationship addiction. These fantasies are part of our early childhood programming, and come from a number of sources, including our parents, romance novels, Hollywood movies, and pornographic magazines. For many of us they are part of a rebellious reaction to our religious upbringings. Whatever the influences, sexual addiction is still an artificial experience created by the mind to escape the fear of intimacy and rejection. When we use sex compulsively, we deny our feelings. Healing comes about when we truly feel our feelings, and embrace all of who we are.

When sex evolves out of love and both partners are totally present with each other, instead of in their fantasies, it can carry them beyond the mind into an experience of merging. It is a source of deep nourishment and fulfillment without attachment. This is the love that many of us are searching for in the singles bars and in our romantic fantasies. This is the love that heals. Somewhere deep within each and every one of us we know that this love is possible, even though we may have forgotten how to reconnect with it.

Saying Yes to Change

Our intuitive voice tells us that the desire for artificial expansion which is at the source of addiction is not really nurturing. Yet because we are surrounded by an addictive society that approves our behavior (just look at the ads on TV), it is easier to ignore our inner voice than to change. One of the many paradoxes of life is that, although change is the natural way of life (as in the change of seasons), we misuse our precious energy in an effort to resist it.

It's as if we are swimming upstream. If only we could let go and float, life would take us on a dynamic journey, more exciting than the one provided by any of the artificial sources of expansion we are currently addicted to. In fact, we probably would no longer desire most of them. Unfortunately, most of us are attached to what seems like a "comfortable" life. We fear changes we don't have control over. We play it safe and stick to what feels "natural" in order to protect ourselves from potential harm or destruction and death. The unfortunate irony is that, if we succeed in accomplishing our goal, we often create a living death.

Change is the only permanent factor in life. It is eternal. Change is life in perpetual motion. It is the dance between contraction and expansion. We don't prefer inhaling over exhaling; why then do we value expansion more than contraction? It seems so unnatural. Go ahead. Try to only inhale for the next ten minutes. It's impossible. If we can accept the cycle of breath as a natural physical phenomenon, what will it take to recognize and accept this basic cycle in the rest of our life as well?

For some it may be a life-threatening illness, for others a life-threatening addiction, for still others a depression that won't go away. Whatever the crisis, it wakes us up to the awareness that our life is not working and we are not living at our maximum potential.

Our attempts to produce expansion artificially after our wake-up call become more and more strained. We begin to experience a more intense source of contraction, a sense of hopelessness. If we listen to our wake-up call it will lead us on a journey inward in search of organic expansion, because the artificial highs no longer seem to be producing the old results.

One of the many paradoxes of healing is that at the beginning of the process we begin to experience moments of expansion through our journey inward, and the simple acceptance of what we discover. As we experience this natural expansion, we begin to let down our guard and release control. As a result, much of the repressed emotional energy that has been stored within our subconscious surfaces. It usually begins with anger, followed by sadness, which is often mislabeled as depression. It is then followed by apathy and discouragement, eventually hitting rock bottom with despair. Then, if we allow ourselves to question and to listen, new choices and new solutions will appear, moving us into creative action. By honoring the natural flow between contraction and expansion, by letting go of our judgments and attachments one by one, we can allow our tears to evolve into laughter.

Healing involves saying yes to all of who we are, including our illness and addiction, our anger and sadness, our fear and denial. As we become interested in the disowned part of ourselves, the part that we have been afraid to look at, we can begin to create an opening for healing. On the healing journey we must travel through the darkness to return to the light.

When we learn to reconnect with ourselves through meditation, we begin to accept the cycle of expansion, which is looking outside of ourselves, and contraction, which is looking within. As we learn to accept the outer circumstances of our lives through seeking, questioning, and observing, we learn to welcome contraction as an opportunity to journey inward. When we take the time to embrace our inner self, and to heal the pain of unfinished business, we can reconnect with the gift of our intuitive wisdom and discover how magnificently simple life is.

15

Embracing
the Child Within

*What is essential is invisible to the eye. It is
only with the heart that one can truly see.*

Antoine Saint-Exupéry,
The Little Prince

WHEN WE ARE BORN, we are each a pure and innocent being,
which I call the soul child. Because our minds are not yet fully
developed, our energy moves naturally between contraction and
expansion without resistance. When our minds are not trying to
control our energy, it can flow between the extreme opposites of
light and dark, as it was designed to do. Our virgin minds do not
yet judge the light as better than the dark.

As we grow, however, we begin to develop a personality, filled
with judgments, usually based on confusing messages from our
parents and teachers. For example, when a child falls and scrapes
her knee, an instinctive natural response is to cry or scream in pain.
Yet often the parent tries to comfort the child because he or she
feels helpless in the face of the child's pain, or guilty that the child
was hurt. If a mother tells a child, "Don't cry. You'll be okay. It's
nothing," she is denying the child's natural reaction. It's as if she
skips a step in an effort to make it better. Even though the child
may be comforted for the moment, she learns to distrust her feelings. She also learns, on a subtle, subconscious level, that pain is
bad, and that something has to be done to make it go away.

It is often a parent's own subconscious judgment regarding

pain that intervenes. Had the mother not been around, for instance, or had she been able simply to allow the child's hurt feelings, the emotional energy would have run its course naturally and the child would be off and playing again. A parent can literally stop the natural unfolding of emotion and begin to limit the natural flow of energy.

Most of us were raised by people who didn't have much freedom, people who therefore imposed all of their restrictive conditioning on us. I'm not suggesting that they were bad. They were doing their best to discipline us, and most likely someone had imposed their conditioning on them when they were young as well. Still, this creates blocks in the natural flow of our emotional energy. If, as children, we had a temper tantrum, for example, or needed to express rage, many of our parents would never let us complete it naturally. Such emotions were considered bad, and at times we were threatened with punishment if we expressed them. Most of our parents didn't give us room to be the emotional beings that we were.

In my own life, whenever I was playing and having fun with my brother, my parents would shout, "Stop it, you're going to hurt yourself. If you don't slow down, you're gonna end up crying." Sure enough, it would happen. Because my energy was free-flowing, it was disturbing to them. They didn't know how to handle the simple joy and celebration of life I was experiencing because they were so uncomfortable with their own feelings.

Before we know it, we learn to behave just like our parents, and we become conditioned beings. Our energy no longer flows naturally, and we begin to repress it in order to fit in. As we grow up, we adapt ourselves to the ways of society as a means of survival. We develop a personality, and we become "good" little girls and boys. We adapt to belong and get what we think we need to be happy: a relationship, a successful career, the right wardrobe, the perfect physique, money in the bank, a car, a fur coat, an exotic trip. Of course, many of these items are useful tools and are not intrinsically bad; it is our greed and attachment to them that is the source of the problem. The personality gets hooked on the system.

It doesn't have much presence without all those attachments to the material world.

In a crisis, the first reaction of the personality is, "What can I do and how can I fix it?" It's a doer. It's a fixer. It's not bad. It's how we go about life. Like sophisticated robots, we do whatever is required to get what we want. We make the money to buy our happiness. If we have a problem, we fix it. We don't take the time to see if the problem is a symptom of something greater. It doesn't occur to us that perhaps the problem is life's way of signaling us. We don't consider it as our wake-up call. We simply congratulate ourselves for solving the problem and escaping one more time. The personality is a master of survival through manipulation and escape.

With each crisis, we become more dependent on outside solutions, and our personality mask becomes bigger. We are less and less vulnerable, and move farther and farther away from our true self, the soul child. The way of the soul is effortless. The way of the personality is often a struggle. The way of the soul is natural. It is divine. It is who we are and why we are alive. It is the way of love.

Healing requires the willingness to reconnect with the inner grace of our soul child. In fact, I believe disease is a cry from the soul, reminding us to live in our hearts and reconnect with the vertical path. When we are faced with the discomfort of disease, surrendering to the anguish and contraction of physical pain can serve as a passage back to the way of the soul.

The Soul Child

It is in the earliest years of our lives that we are closest to living the life of the soul. There's nothing we need to do, all of our basic needs are taken care of (except of course in the case of an abused or neglected baby). In this state of innocence and bliss we have nothing to hide. We openly celebrate the joy of our being. We play and laugh and cry with equal intensity, flowing with the dance of contraction and expansion. Our minds are empty and new. The universe is a magical mystery to us. Every day is a miracle.

The energy of this child still lives within us today, although most of us disregard it. It is truly one of the saddest aspects about growing up: the unconscious disconnection that is created when we leave the soul child in us behind in order to adapt to our community. Some of you may have worked in various workshops and therapies on accessing this part of yourself, also called the magical child. She/he is a wonderful source of joy and inspiration, a free spirit who shares love unconditionally. Had our childhoods been a safe place to be ourselves, perhaps we might not have abandoned this part of us. What a wonderful world it will be when we learn to trust our soul child again and live from our hearts.

As young children, we quickly sense the fear and hypocrisy around us. Because it contradicts our own innocent sense of compassion and honesty, we question why some of us are starving while others have plenty to eat. We question why people inflict pain and hurt on one another just because they look different. We wonder why the world is not more fair, and why we can't all play together. We question why there has to be fighting, and war and killing. Yet our innocent questions are ignored, or answered dishonestly, and we begin to feel that something is intrinsically wrong with us.

The Adapted Child Survivor

The reason we automatically adapt from the natural path of the soul to the conditional path of the personality is because it is the only way we know how to survive. When we are born, we are helpless infants depending solely on our parents for survival. Approval feels like love, and disapproval feels like the removal of love. Our parents' love is of the utmost importance to us. Without it we would literally die, since we are helpless infants unable to care for ourselves.

We quickly discover that if we smile a certain way at Daddy we are rewarded with cuddles and kisses, yet if we play with our feces, he frowns. We learn that if we cry long and hard enough Mommy will feed us, yet if we throw our food around Mommy will take it away. Suddenly we have some kind of control over our destiny. We discover that if we behave a certain way Mommy and Daddy will love us, but if we behave in another way, even if it feels natural, they won't. Of course our parents don't actually remove their love; they believe they are teaching children proper behavior, but their shift in energy feels like a withholding of love. Our survival instinct is so strong that we quickly learn to adapt ourselves in order to maintain our parents' love. Because of our instinct to survive, we eventually adapt ourselves to the ways of the world, betraying our own childlike hearts.

Children are so sensitive to energy that they immediately pick up the negative vibrations from their parents' judgments, lies, and disapproval. They also quickly become aware of the dishonesty and hypocrisy between adults. They can tell Mommy is upset even if she is speaking words to the contrary. Children learn hypocrisy when they hear Daddy say he'll be home to tuck them in, only to find that, due to his late work schedule, they have to go to bed without his goodnight kiss. They learn to adapt to lies and broken promises. In fact, they learn to lie as well. The child who innocently breaks something may lie as a form of self-protection in response to a parent's threatening accusation. The child fears that if he were to admit the truth, Daddy might stop loving him and then he would not survive.

Again, this fear of death is a real response to a very real survival threat. If we were to be abandoned as infants, we would die. Fortunately, our bodies and minds develop so that we can learn to take care of ourselves. Unfortunately, we also develop a package of conditioning which influences our every action, and a set of beliefs which act as filters through which we perceive our reality. One of the strongest of these filters is the belief that we are unworthy.

Our Fall from Eden

As we are forced by the circumstances of our life to adapt ourselves, we detach slowly but surely from the true feelings of our heart. We compromise ourselves to gain or maintain the love that we know, on a soul level, we deserve. Naturally we love the people around us unconditionally, and unnaturally that love is returned conditionally. This creates our first sense of unworthiness.

Every time we deny our inner truth in order to fit in, we program a permanent subconscious decision into our minds, a belief that the world is not a safe place to express who we truly are. We begin to view the world through the filter of mistrust, and develop a defense system to protect our soul child. Because we have lost touch with our innate sense of trust, we control, judge, and manipulate the world around us to get our needs met.

It is in this moment that we shift from the energy of human beings to that of human doings. This is what the fall from Eden symbolizes. Original sin is the direct result of our turning away from God, and mistrusting the perfect flow of the universe. This fall from grace usually happens by the time we are four years old. By then we have learned the ways of the world and the tricks of the trade.

As we begin to become more autonomous, we continue to use our tricks to get our needs met. We live in the constant cycle of desire. We experience expansion when our needs are fulfilled and contraction when we fear that our needs will be unmet. This is when we begin to seek artificial sources of expansion, to run from the fear which plagues us: *If my desires are not fulfilled I will die.* Even though our basic needs of food, water, air, and shelter are taken care of, we still feel in need. In our adapted programming, we perceive the expansion we feel through desire fulfillment as love, which the child in us equates with survival.

This is because we are no longer connected to the natural grace of expansion and bliss we experienced as a soul child. That bliss, which is a source of healing, can exist only in the innocence of our beingness. This innocence, like healing, is an allowing, not a doing; we cannot make it happen. All we can do is create an opening for it by letting go of control (the urge to make life the way we think it should be) and opening ourselves to what is available in the moment.

PROCESS

Dialogue with Your Soul Child

(Read the entire process first before doing it.)

Create a safe, private environment in a room where you will not be disturbed by anyone or anything, including the telephone. Sit in a comfortable position on your bed or on the floor and place a pillow or cushion in front of you, leaving approximately two feet between the cushion and yourself. If it is more comfortable, you may use two chairs, facing each other, placing the pillow on the chair in front of you.

With open eyes, simply observe your breath as you inhale and exhale. Begin to rub your thighs gently, and feel yourself sitting in the room. Become aware of your physical surroundings, including the temperature of the room, and any sounds or smells that may be around you. Let yourself be aware of the current circumstances of your life, as well as your resistance to them. Just observe yourself, no need to judge. Simply be present, in the moment, with all its fullness of circumstances, emotions, and reactions. Take your time to watch the entire process of the flow of your thoughts as they continuously change.

Allow your mind to slow down, and simply let yourself be. Spend two to three minutes watching the process of your mind. Observe how you feel right now. Are you sitting on a volcano of emotions? Are you anxious? Are you afraid? Are you uncomfortable? Simply watch your feelings about sitting alone in the room. Notice how much energy it requires to stay focused on what is happening right now. Simply allow yourself to be there, watching yourself breathe and rubbing your thighs. Allow your train of thoughts to simply be there as well, without engaging in them. If you do engage in them, simply return to observing your breath. You are now experiencing the state I call the present adult. This is the capable part of you who is able to provide food, shelter, and clothing for yourself. He/she exists only in the present moment.

Once you feel you are present, imagine yourself as a young child, sitting in front of you on the cushion. Trust that your subconscious will provide you with the right image of yourself. You might not have a clear picture; do not let that stop you. It will be enough if you just have a feeling of the soul child inside of you.

When you are ready, begin your dialogue in your own way. You might start simply by saying "Hello, how are you?" and then inviting your soul child to share whatever she is feeling with you. Then physically switch seats and sit on the cushion in front of you and close your eyes.

Let yourself become that very young, innocent child. Let yourself sink into the experience of being her. Feel her pure joy for life, her curiosity, her awe, and her endless questions. Let yourself experience life as fresh and new, perhaps being puzzled by the behavior of the adults around you. Perhaps you cannot understand why people are hungry or homeless, or why people are killing each other.

Allow yourself to spend time in that pure, innocent energy, so closely connected to our collective soul. Allow yourself to share your feelings with your present adult. Feel the love, gratitude, and trust as well as your genuine desire to share. Feel how relaxed your body is, and how accepting of yourself you are, just because you are alive. Breathe and rejoice.

If a question arises, verbally ask it of your present adult. Then physically switch back to your original seat, and open your eyes. Allow yourself to return to the awareness of the here and now, feeling yourself in the capable adult body of your present circumstances. With total honesty, allow yourself to respond to your soul child. When you respond, let it be from the simplicity of the present moment, which is always new, open, and vulnerable. Avoid the tendency to respond from the past, with all of its judgments and control. For example, you may simply say: "I hear you. Thank you for sharing," or "I understand that you don't want to talk right now, and that's all right. I appreciate your honesty." In the now, you may not know too much more than what you are receiving from your senses in that moment. Follow your heart, and share what you are feeling, in response to your soul child's sharing. It may be gratitude, compassion, or sadness. Let yourself be surprised.

Now allow yourself to switch seats again and close your eyes. Let your soul child speak again, perhaps in response to what you just said, or anything else that may be coming up for him or her. Don't censor anything, just allow it to be expressed as is. Continue the dialogue, switching seats back and forth as you switch roles, until the soul child feels complete for now. When you finish the dialogue, finish as the present adult. It is extremely important always to begin and end the dialogue in the reality of the present adult.

Healing Versus Survival

Having our life threatened by a stigmatic disease like AIDS automatically throws us into survival mode. In this state of emergency, our minds are desperately trying to find a solution. Unfortunately, our usual solutions come from the strategies of the child survivor, designed to avoid deeper fear and pain. Rarely do they produce the expected results of healing.

In the healing process, it is important to slow down and connect with the creativity of our soul child, which is a doorway to our healer within. Healing can occur when we balance the restrictive path of survival with the naturally flowing path of the soul. Of course this is easier said than done. When we are panicking about our survival, it can be very difficult to stay connected to the way of the soul.

Reconnecting with the soul child is only half the process of healing the inner child. It is also very important to work with the child that we have become, the adapted child survivor. The soul child and the child survivor are two facets of the same energy. They are a twin energy in us. The soul child responds with enthusiasm to the challenges of life, while the child survivor uses all her intelligence and energy to find short cuts, unaware that they are illusions.

We have spent the majority of our life disconnected from the purity and innocence of our soul child, relying more on the child survivor, because he is a master at coping with the circumstances of our life. There is a beauty and innocence in the faithful perseverance of the child survivor, who constantly tries to protect the soul child from harm, but it mostly keeps us from growing. When the same perseverance is in the hands of the present adult, we have the freedom to create change in our lives.

Meeting Our Child Survivor

Inside each of us is a frightened and vulnerable child in need of love. She is afraid of rejection and abandonment, because she is afraid of death. She is angry at the abuse she has had to bear, and at all the broken promises she has had to endure. She is sad about her lost innocence, and the emptiness and loneliness she feels inside. Because she has been hurt so much she is afraid to live.

This dark side of us is so repressed that for all intents and purposes she has been abandoned. Unfortunately, the more we run from her the more she runs us. This child within is precious and lovable when we consciously nurture her, but left alone she will do anything to avoid pain and death, including creating disease.

As we approach our healing, moving through resistance and denial, feelings that have been repressed begin to bubble up to the surface. These are the feelings we may not have had room to express as children, so we stuffed them away in neat little packages, using tremendous energy to keep those emotions under control.

By the time we are adolescents we have stored a whole pack-

age of repressed emotions within us. As we move farther and farther away from the balance of opposites, we lose our ability to
trust the flow of the cycle. We limit our capacity to expand naturally because of our constant evaluation of life as either good or
bad. We become attached to expansion because "it feels good,"
and we avoid contraction because it doesn't.

As adults, most of us are walking around with our packages
filled with what we consider to be negative emotions: fear, anger,
sadness, parts of ourselves that we judge as too painful to look at.
Perhaps we fear that if we were to open the package and finally give
expression to those repressed feelings, we may lose control. Unfortunately it is the part of us that controls that created the repression in the first place. Eventually the package will explode on its
own. Healing involves making a conscious choice to allow this
explosion to happen as part of a healthy expression of feelings in
a safe environment.

Subconscious Decisions about Life

While growing up we made personal vows that still rule our present
life. Decisions like "The world is not a safe place," "I will never let
anyone love me or hurt me again," or "I am not worthy." Most of
these decisions about life were based on the idea of being good,
originating from the fear that we could not survive on our own.

These decisions happened on a subconscious level. Parents
know how to manipulate their children through positive and negative attitudes. The source of all notions of "good" and "bad"
basically start on this subconscious level. Because these decisions
were made on the subconscious level, it is very useful to become
aware of our primary decisions and their hidden variations.

As children, we knew that rejection by our parents was the
most life-threatening circumstance in our universe, to be avoided at
any cost. It is then imperative for us as adults challenged by a
life-threatening illness to recognize the impact these decisions still
have on our physical body. It is also vital to recognize how much
the child survivor can cripple the present adult.

Healing those subconscious decisions is brought about by returning to the event that was the source of the decision to be a powerless victim. In my personal life and in therapy sessions with most of my clients, this means returning to a series of traumatic events in early childhood, which becomes intensified during adolescence, and which often is magnified to its maximum degree in our adulthood. The event might have appeared insignificant to those who were around the child at the time of the event, but for the young child it literally registered as a life-threatening moment.

Traumatic Childhood Events

An example of this is a situation in which a mother threatens to leave her young child forever if he does not stop crying. She knows very well that she is using one of her "tools" to obtain the behavior she wants from the child, but because the child lives totally in the moment, he literally fears for his life when the door of his room closes and his mother disappears. The child has no notion of the probability of his mother returning, and because the intensity of his fear of not surviving is so violent, a deep sense of victimization is embedded in his consciousness. Because the child literally cannot live without his mother's love and nourishment, from that moment on he will make a vow to avoid any situation that reminds him of that frightening experience of abandonment.

A child does not have a context for understanding the withdrawal of love. Because she perceives herself as the center of her universe, she interprets every disruption of love personally. A baby needs love and care from her parents, not only in the form of security, food, and shelter, but also because when a baby is first born she does not yet comprehend her physical separation from the light and love of the source. For example, a child is bonded with her mother not only on the physical level, through the need for sustenance and security, but also on the soul level. A baby's connection with her mother goes very deep, because a mother is the passageway from the light and love of the source, to this world.

While an infant's mind is still pure, she is living totally from the heart. When a child first arrives in this world, she is still connected with the eternal, and often the adults around her become reconnected with what is eternal in them. It is usually a moment of deep grace. When a doctor separates a baby from her mother at birth and stores her in a room away from her most important connection, the infant loses the vital energy of the heart and is rapidly exposed to the survival energy of the mind.

The infant is then subjected to the various procedures that someone has intellectually assumed will be best for her, but are usually quite unnatural. For instance, who on earth can prove that feeding a baby every three hours is good for her, when her natural cycle might be every two hours? Because of this fixed schedule, she may have to wait one full hour in misery, and experience it as a traumatic event that could take a lifetime to heal.

Because of these events and the decisions we make as a result of them—such as "I am helpless" or "I am not good enough"—we live in a chronic state of self-denial and self-doubting. These decisions form a prison guarded by our inner child's need for outer approval. He or she may wear many masks to hide the sense of shame and escape the fear of abandonment, but those feelings still influence every aspect of our lives.

It is very important to understand the decisions we have made while growing up, and to realize that they are no longer valid. Most of the time we are not even aware that as full-grown adults we are still reacting to and rebelling against our parents. We are also unaware of the full consequences of those decisions.

P R O C E S S

Dialogue with Our Child Survivor

(Read the entire process first before doing it.)

Healing through self-mastery is available when we return to the event that is the source of the disempowering life decision that we are helpless victims and release the emotions related to it. Dialogue with the child survivor is one effective way to achieve this.

Again place a pillow in front of you and sit on the floor, or on your bed (or use two chairs, placing the pillow on the chair facing you). You are now in your present adult. Keep your eyes open and become aware of what is now. Bring your focus to the present by connecting with the physical sensations in and around you. Tune in to your body. Become aware of your breath as you inhale and exhale. Feel your heartbeat. Touch your thighs. Feel your clothing against your skin. If there is any pain or tension in your body, simply witness it without judgment. Become aware of your physical surroundings: the temperature of the room, and any sounds or smells that may be around you. Do whatever you can to bring your awareness into the here and now.

Once you feel you have arrived and are totally present, imagine yourself as a child sitting in the chair facing you. Again, trust your subconscious to provide you with the right image of your child survivor. If you have difficulty visualizing him then just tune in to the way he feels.

When you feel ready, ask this imaginary child what he is afraid of, or angry or sad about. Invite the child to share with you what he is feeling. Now switch seats, and close your eyes.

Allow yourself to become your child survivor. Let your body language and voice change, and verbally express your feelings out loud. Don't edit anything. Just let your stream of consciousness as the child survivor flow uninterrupted. Allow whatever emotions may arise, such as anger and sadness, to be expressed.

Perhaps you will feel lost and puzzled, or want love from someone from whom you are not able to get it. Perhaps you will experience the frustration of not being understood, or of not understanding someone else, even though you may be trying very hard. Maybe you will feel emotional pain at the loss of unconditional love. Notice what survival tools you immediately think of as a way to get that love back. Notice what decisions you made about life—that life is not fair, that love is too painful, or that you will never let yourself be hurt again. Let yourself remember when you first began to receive the negative message that something was wrong with you.

Let yourself express whatever emotion comes up. Let the tears or the anger flow. Let your emotional release heal whatever core decisions stand in your way because your child survivor did not feel safe at the time to express his feelings. Let yourself complete the unfinished business and finally express your feelings. Allow yourself to finally say out loud the things you were not allowed to say at the time, but which you are still carrying with you.

Let yourself heal your emotions about the fact that you were forced to become a survivor and adapt yourself to a defensive, aggressive, and suspicious world. Your child might feel a deep pain at the loss of that innate trust he once had, which has been violated so many times. Notice the powerful core decision you made at that time.

Let your child survivor finish expressing whatever he feels. In the beginning, he may not want to say anything. He may not trust you yet. That's okay. He may want to blame, judge, complain to, or manipulate you. He may be very angry. When the child seems complete for the moment, or asks you a question, switch back to your original seat, and open your eyes.

Allow yourself to refocus on the reality of the now. Again, when you respond to the child, let it be from the simplicity of the present moment, which is always new, open, and vulnerable. Avoid the tendency to respond from the past, with all of its judgments and control. Avoid the urge to play an authoritarian parental role, giving advice or trying to change the way the child is feeling. Just be there for the child in a caring, supportive manner, simply from what is now.

In the present moment, you may not know too much more than what you are receiving from your senses right now. You may feel gratitude for the child's willingness to share, or compassion for his inability to trust. If he was distrustful, tell him that it is okay. Explain to him that you understand and ask him if he wants to talk about why he feels that way. It is important to accept whatever the child expresses, including anger and silence. Follow your heart, and share with compassion your response to the child's sharing, so that he will feel safe enough eventually to open up.

When you have finished, ask your child if he has anything else to share. Then switch seats again and close your eyes. Let your child speak again, perhaps in response to what you just said, or about anything else that may be coming up for him. Again, don't censor, just allow him to release his pent-up feelings. Continue the dialogue, switching seats as you switch roles, until the child feels complete; then finish as the present adult self. Again, it is very important to always begin and end the dialogue in the present moment.

When you are back in the present adult, you may want to take your child (the cushion) in your arms and embrace him. Allow both of you to experience this reunion, of finding each other, feeling the gratitude for the deep honesty and simple communication between the two of you. Comfort him if he needs reassurance that you will always be there for him; assure him that he is safe in your arms and that you will take care of him. Allow yourself to experience the embrace for as long as you want, and then gently open your eyes at your own pace.

Here is a sample dialogue to use as a guideline. Remember, it is only a guideline. There is no "right" way for the child survivor to respond.

As you sit in the present, watching your breath, allow yourself to sink into the warm compassion of your heart and invite your child to share with you. Remember to listen without judgment.

PRESENT ADULT Hey little one, what would you like to talk about?

CHILD SURVIVOR I don't really want to talk to you. You are always telling me what to do, and how to do it. That makes me angry. [Pauses and is silent.]

P.A. [Remember to reconnect with the energy of acceptance before you respond to the child. He might have simply been testing you to see if you are really giving him the space to express himself.] I understand your feelings, but for now I promise you that I will not try to make you do anything. If you like, we can talk about how it makes you feel when you are told what to do, and when to do it. Would you like that?

C.S. Yes, but I want to talk without you interrupting me.

P.A. [Take a deep breath.] Okay, I can do that.

C.S. You don't respect me. You are just like my mother. You are always correcting me, and always telling me what to do, and most of all always interrupting me when I am really beginning to have fun. Every time I begin to laugh, you come rushing in with something serious to do that has to be done right away. It is not true. Nothing is more important than having fun and being happy and I am really pissed off at you for taking that away from me.

P.A. I understand. That would upset me too.

C.S. Really? They why do you make us do that? I really don't understand, you are just like Mom.

P.A. Tell me what you feel about Mom.

C.S. Oh, she makes me so angry. I hate her, she never lets me play with my toys. They always have to be kept in order in the closet. Why do I have them, if I cannot play with them? And we can never have friends either. We never have friends coming and playing with us. I feel so lonely.

P.A. I am sorry to hear that you are lonely, but right now I am with you, and believe it or not, I am a friend too. If you show me how, maybe we can play together.

C.S. I'd like that.

P.A. Thank you so much for telling me that. I don't know very much how to have fun, but I definitely am willing to try. You made such a good point. From now on I will show you what is fun over here, in my world. It may be a bit different than your toys and games, but they are really fun too. Would you like that?

C.S. Maybe. As long as you don't go too fast. You often go so fast. But yes I'd like to play with your toys. My toys sometimes are boring.

P.A. [Embracing the pillow in your arms] Thank you so much for being so honest with me. I appreciate you, and I love you very much. I promise I will never let you down. I am here for you, to be your friend. Together we can discover how to have fun.

Write down in your journal whatever core decisions you remembered making at an early age and the feelings you still have about them. Also list anything else that may seem important (for instance, key fears, issues of anger or sadness, or the fact that he was not willing to talk today) so that you can begin a dialogue with the child about that specific issue at a later time, and continue the healing process.

This will help you to understand that those core decisions were made with the limited viewpoint of a young child. He could not be aware of all the elements involved, nor of any extenuating circumstances. These decisions may have been appropriate at the time, but they no longer are.

This dialogue can be practiced daily as a way to get to know your child survivor. It also can serve you whenever you feel contracted—in fear or anger, for example. You can begin to heal that wounded child within by having a dialogue with him and slowly bringing him more and more into your present reality. As you demonstrate to your child that you are now in charge of your life, you can begin to re-parent yourself as the capable adult that you now are.

Sample Questions

Here is a list of some sample questions you may want to ask your child survivor as a way to begin your daily dialogues. Feel free to express the questions in your own words, addressing the question in a sober way, and as directly as you can.

1. What do you feel about this disease?
2. What do you feel about our doctor?
3. What do you feel about our present treatments?
4. Why are you confused?
5. What do you feel about death?
6. What do you feel about the way we live right now?
7. What do you feel about our relationship with our lover?
8. What do you feel about Mommy?
9. What do you feel about Daddy?
10. What would you like to learn?
11. What is your heart longing for?
12. Do you trust me?
13. How is your connection with me?
14. What do you want to tell me that you haven't in a long time?
15. What are you angry about?
16. What are you sad about?
17. What are you afraid of?
18. What makes you happy?
19. What do you wanna do for fun?
20. How can I take better care of you?

16

Survival Masks
of the Child

*There is love, that is the same all over the
world. . . . And unless we have the elements of love dominating this entire exhi-
bition, we better take it down before we
put it up.*

—EDWARD STEICHEN

WHEN WE are challenged by life, we attempt to deal with it with
the limited survival tools of a four-year-old child. These tools include lying, seducing, manipulating, withdrawing, running away,
and having a temper tantrum. As adults, we may wear sophisticated masks and play a variety of roles to disguise our tactics, but
we are still using the same survival tools we developed as helpless
infants. These masks, which include those of the victim, the judge,
the controller, and the indulger, comprise our personality.

These various aspects of our personality try the best they can
to cope with what they perceive as life-threatening events, such as
episodes of fear, rejection, and criticism. At times they serve a
useful purpose, yet they do not know how to heal, only how to
survive. In fact, some of these very masks are responsible for pro-
moting dis-ease in the first place.

These masks were created when we were very young, as a way
to survive in the outside world. We developed these aspects of our
personality because the world did not always appear to be a safe
place for us, or because our parents were not always able to provide us with the love and nurturing we needed.

The Masks of Personality

Most of us believe that we *are* our personalities with their many masks. It's as if the masks we are wearing are so close to our faces that we have forgotten we have them on. These masks or subpersonalities are our child survivor's defense mechanisms for dealing with our daily life. They are also the part of us responsible for coping with crises as they arise.

The child survivor changes masks constantly, adapting to life's circumstances with the agility of a magician. The mask of the judge might evolve into the controller, then into the people-pleaser, then into the know-it-all. In this chameleonlike existence, it is extremely difficult to discover who we really are *behind* the masks.

For example, let's examine the strategy of the child survivor in doing what she does best, which is avoiding pain. In order to avoid pain, or create a superficial sense of pleasure, the child survivor chooses an action. At first she is very excited, but as she thinks about it she realizes that the action could cause pain. She then rethinks her tactics and brings forth the mask of the controller, whose job it is to protect the child. He warns, you might get hurt, so don't do it. Escape. So next appears the saboteur, who will stop the motion toward the goal, perhaps through an accident. If she succeeds in sabotaging the goal, the child dons the mask of the complainer to justify her action and enroll others into her predicament with the hope of getting a lot of recognition and agreement.

When we are in a complainer mode, we set the stage for the mask of the victim, which is a very popular one. We can get a lot of attention with that mask, through our "poor me" attitude. The child then confuses the attention she is getting with the love she craves. She can justify not taking any action in the first place, and feel good about it. This keeps her in the victim role, and makes her believe in the mask so totally that she is no longer aware of the mechanism.

Outdated Survival Programs

Healing can happen when we realize that we are more than just our personality, which is based on the survival programs of a four-year-old child. This realization permits us to access the present adult in us, who is fully capable of discovering creative solutions to life crises.

Most of us are walking around with outdated subconscious survival programs telling us that we are not safe and that it is not okay to be open, honest, and vulnerable. For example, a decision that many of us have programmed for ourselves equates love with pain: "If I let myself love again, I will be rejected and hurt." The programming concludes that if I am rejected, "I will die."

These subconscious programs, based on the literal life-threatening events of a helpless infant, are no longer relevant or appropriate to the capable adults that most of us are today. Yet, even though the majority of us are leading full, successful lives, the old subconscious programs still filter our perceptions. They keep us in a constant state of emergency, resulting in high anxiety and stress.

Because these masks are old defense mechanisms developed in response to events of childhood, when we were actually helpless, it is important to help the inner child feel safe today. When we do so, she is then able to blossom and express herself openly with spontaneous joy. It may take several dialogues with the child, with repeated reassurances that she is safe with you, before she will begin to trust again.

The first step in healing the inner child is the willingness to look within and say hello to that vulnerable part of ourselves, and to all the masks of survival the child wears. This step leads to a letting go of judgment and control, and eventually lets us learn how to say yes to who we are and to life as it unfolds. By doing this we are learning to say yes creatively to the present circumstances of our life. This promotes healing energy instead of defensive survival energy.

The reason it is so important to recognize and engage in dialogue with all the different masks that the child survivor wears is not to make them wrong, but to understand their direct opposition to the soul child and the healer. After all, the child survivor wants the same things that the soul child and the healer want, which is simply to love and be loved. When we realize this, we can begin to reparent ourselves in a mature and appropriate way, finally giving ourselves permission fully to be who we are.

The Judge

When we are presented with something disagreeable in our lives, the part of us that wants it to be different is the survival mask of the judge. She judges the people and circumstances of our life, as well as our own vulnerable child.

The job of this mask is to evaluate a person or situation and determine if it will serve us or harm us. If a person or situation is judged as good, the child survivor will want more of it and might even believe that her survival depends on it. If a person or situation is judged as bad, the child survivor will do the opposite, using all of her survival tools to avoid it.

Unfortunately, our judgments about what is good and what is bad are still based on the old survival programs of a helpless infant. Subsequently we move through life reacting to projected fantasies instead of what is actually happening in the moment.

The Judge as a Useful Tool As designed by nature, the judge serves a useful purpose. It is the part of our mind that learns from our mistakes. If as a child we burn our hand touching a hot stove, the judge will remind us of this each time we are near a hot stove, as a way to protect us from getting burned again.

The judge serves a functional purpose in terms of day-to-day living, since it is the part of our mind that determines what is real. For example, without our judge we would not be able to determine whether or not a particular object is a chair before we sit in it, or if a particular substance is edible before we eat it.

Filters of Perception Unfortunately, the program of our judge keeps us a prisoner of our past mistakes and decisions, and limits our ability to live in the present moment. When we perceive life through the filter of the judge, based on the conditioning of a helpless child, our "present moment" is colored by the programming of the past. Therefore we bring a whole package of old perceptions and decisions to every person and every situation we encounter.

This creates unnecessary fear and leads to a reactive instead of a creative way of living. The world of the survivor is reactive, in the sense that we believe life *is done to* us. The world of the healer is creative, in that we are fully responsible for the choices we make in our life.

The Judge Versus the Present Adult Healing involves becoming aware of the voice of the judge within us and consciously choosing whether or not the judgment is still relevant to our lives today. This requires that we discover and access a very conscious part of ourselves, one that does not judge, but merely observes what is. This part of us is the present adult or the "witness." It exists only in the now. (Like when I was baking muffins, and asking the question "What is now?")

Because one of the tactics of the judge is to wear the mask of the present adult as a way of maintaining control, this process can be very tricky. The judge often sounds like our mother, father, or any other adult who played a significant role in our lives. Meditation serves as a powerful tool to assist us in determining the difference in energy between the judge and the present adult.

It is also helpful to examine the other masks that the child survivor wears in tandem with the judge.

The Controller

Some of the other survival tools we use when we are challenged with a life crisis are control, denial, and resistance. The controller is the part of us that wants life to be free from pain as a way to protect the vulnerable child. The controller rejects the way life is happening in the moment because of some picture or idea from the judge prescribing how life "should" be. The controller limits our behavior and our ability to say yes to each moment as it unfolds. Saying no to life is our way of being in control. When we are in control, the child within us feels safe, as if nothing bad can happen to him or her.

We think this protection is necessary because we perceive the world to be separate from us. Its vastness intimidates us. In our fear we seek to control our environment. History is filled with stories of one nation conquering another; men subjugating women; humans harnessing and exploiting animals; and the human species destroying our planet while trying to control nature. When we don the mask of the controller, we slowly become disloyal to life itself.

Avoidance Through Control Control is also a subtle form of avoidance. By trying to control the circumstances and people in my life, I refused to take responsibility for my condition. This kind of control easily leads to blame and denial, survival masks that the child wears to escape from fear. By hiding behind our controller, the child survivor can live in denial indefinitely, feeling as if everything is fine. Unfortunately, this illusion then enables us to avoid taking responsibility for changing the attitude or behavior which is the source of the disease.

When I first started having symptoms, I was not aware of how much my controller was not allowing me to hear the message that my body was sending me. She was doing her job of protecting my vulnerable child from what she feared most, namely sickness and death.

The Controller Versus the Healer When the symptoms increased to the point where I could no longer deny them, the intuitive voice of my inner healer offered me guidance. The healer within, which is closely related to the soul child, recommended that I end my relationship with Nado, ask for emotional support from friends, and express my repressed feelings. Fearing the repercussions, the controller resisted. Using a smoke screen of excuses, the controller denied that anything was wrong. Because I was trusting my controller instead of my healer, the indulger stepped in and I went back to doing whatever felt familiar and comfortable. I basically reverted to the old behavior that promoted the disease to begin with.

The controller is the nemesis of the healer, whose path is trust, acceptance, and surrender. It is important to identify the controller in our lives so that we can consciously choose, moment by moment, to let go of control. This creates a self-discipline that allows healing. Control and discipline may appear the same but they have a very different impact. Control is restrictive and repressive, while discipline is expansive and promotes freedom.

For example, I instinctively knew that I needed to let go of the attitudes I held toward the circumstances of my life. Even though I struggled to change my attitudes, I was usually paralyzed by the fear of not being able to "do it right" and meet the standards of the judge. Instead of simply letting my life unfold, I kept trying to control every moment. In an attempt to avoid what my vulnerable child intensely feared, I used all of my energy to deny it. As I let go and learned to trust my process moment by moment, my self-discipline emerged naturally, and I found I didn't have to force myself to "do the right thing."

Denial

Some of the tools of the controller are the defense mechanisms of denial, resistance, and guilt. Denial is directly related to control. Both control and denial are generated by a belief that life is done to us, that we are victims rather than co-creators of our life. When we are in denial, we may try to control others and whatever circumstances we can around us in an effort to avoid our feelings of helplessness and rage.

Denial as a Useful Tool As I shared in my description of my own healing journey, denial serves an initial positive purpose as a buffer period, but if it is indulged for too long it can ultimately become destructive. For example, when we receive news of some shocking event, such as the loss of a loved one, or our own diagnosis, our first response, is "No!" It is completely natural to reject bad news at first. It is as instinctive as sneezing.

For many of us, it is our only way of coping. How human it is, after all, to deny our condition, at least during the initial adjustment period. When I received my diagnosis, the rug was completely pulled out from underneath me: the bottom fell out. I was stranded, totally numb, not knowing what to do or how to feel. The buffer period of denial allowed me time to integrate the news and its impact on my life.

Denial in Others I can't emphasize enough how important that buffer period was for me. I invite you to give your loved ones and patients time to integrate their diagnoses into their lives. Bear in mind that what may appear to be denial may simply be their attempt to maintain a basic level of dignity.

This can be very difficult for us as friends, relatives, and caregivers, but when we try to help others "overcome" their denial, it only creates resistance. Denial in others activates our own sense of helplessness. It is important to realize that our need to fix the situation is often a response to our own feelings of helplessness. When we deal with someone in denial, it is best to give them room to move out of it naturally, on their own. Simple love and acceptance of where they are and where we are is the most effective tool to support healing.

Denial Through Will One of the forms of denial that I frequently encounter in clients who have just been diagnosed with AIDS is, "I won't die from AIDS." Unlike "I don't have AIDS," this denial is considered a healthy response by caregivers and patients alike. I, on the other hand, see it as potentially destructive, and as an unnecessary source of contraction and stress. The energy it takes to sustain this sort of denial could be used toward healing if the patients would be willing to let go and trust the natural flow of their lives.

In this response, fear and denial are mixed. The fear of facing despair is so strong that a contraction similar to a mental paralysis takes place; the automatic survival system takes over, in the form of "I will not die from this." This defense system creates a strong energy that may drive us for a little while; but like all energy coming from contraction, it will eventually run out. It has been my experience that anything done from the standpoint of will power eventually fails when exhaustion of the will sets in and self-indulgence takes over.

If we acknowledge that denial is a perfectly normal reaction, as part of a complex set of reactions, including resistance, fear, guilt, etc., it will make it much easier to move through this stage. Saying yes to denial in advance allows healing to happen more quickly and sets up a healthier relationship with those aspects of ourselves that we are denying.

Resistance

If denial is putting up a temporary barrier to our feelings as a way of coping with shock and pain, resistance is the hardening of that barrier into a permanent wall. That wall protects us from the pain of our contraction, but also limits us from experiencing the joy of our expansion. Brick by brick we cut ourselves off from our feelings. Living in resistance, saying no to our lives as they are presented to us, obstructs our natural energy from flowing and provides a fertile breeding ground for disease.

After denial begins to wear off, resistance is the next defense mechanism that the child survivor uses to cope with crisis. Unfortunately, the more we resist what we fear, the more real we make it. It's like the old saying, "What we resist, persists."

Resistance is also another form of control. When our energy seeks to flow in one direction and we resist it, we restrict it from flowing at all. When we resist our natural emotional response to a crisis, we also restrict the natural healing energy within us.

Resistance as a Useful Tool Resistance can have a positive side as well, and it is related to this restriction of energy. Much discomfort builds up when we resist what life is offering us, and eventually the awareness of the need for personal transformation becomes painfully evident. The tension we generate through resistance is like the discomfort of holding our breath before we cry or scream. We cannot remain in the position of resistance for very long without expending more and more energy. When we become aware that we are resisting, the energy that has been accumulated can be released like a spring, propelling us into acceptance.

When we are finally willing to accept our condition and feel our pain, we can begin to let down our resistance. This is the first step of healing; simple acceptance of what is. When we are willing to admit that we are sick and presently powerless over the situation, healing can begin. As we find the courage to admit our feelings, we discover the strength to express them. As we release the emotional energy repressed inside, resistance begins to melt away and we create an opening for healing.

Self-Denial

If we remain in our resistance for too long it can generate another more destructive form of denial, namely self-denial. When I look at the pattern of resistance throughout my life, I see that the source of it is a deep fear of being who I know I am. Although in my heart I am in touch with the master within me, I am unable to fully integrate it into my life. This is because my past is filled with numerous incidents when I found it too difficult to assert myself, or to speak my truth with others. Those painful memories somehow seem more real than those rare moments when I did act from the master that I am. Allowing the past to limit my experience of the present is another example of how I resist standing up for who I am. It is another way to indulge the victim in me.

Our society prefers that individuals remain powerless and do not wake up to become masters of themselves. If too many of us were to take charge of our own lives, then the governments and religions could no longer control us. In that event, society would naturally evolve into a healthy, autonomous community. Each member would assume full responsibility for his or her participation in a commonly shared society.

In an effort to control that evolution and maintain the status quo, those in power make the world of the victim very appealing to the masses. We receive a lot more social validation and emotional "strokes" as victims than as masters, so it is the more popular choice. To live from true self-mastery takes a lot of discipline.

Self-Denial Is a Dis-ease

Self-denial is a dis-ease unto itself and has affected most of us in one form or another. We have disowned and denied a part of ourselves for so long, it feels almost natural. Growing up in dysfunctional families, we have had to constantly deny who we are to keep the peace, or to avoid being beaten. In school we deny who we are in effort to fit in. In relationships we hide the part of us we judge harshly, so that people will like us, and then we judge ourselves as unworthy when they leave. We repress our emotions, and hide our shame. We blame ourselves, and then feel guilty about it. We go on diets and join gyms to change our bodies, buy new wardrobes and hold status jobs to mask the unworthiness we feel inside.

This is the real dis-ease that needs healing. It is the greatest plague of our time. It's much like a genetic illness handed down from generation to generation. We poison our children unknowingly because we are unaware of how sick we are. It's time to discover where this sickness comes from, how we perpetuate it, and who we really are as healthy beings.

Self-denial can take many forms, including addiction, abuse, and destructiveness. It originates from a deep sense of unworthiness. The core decision that "I'm not good enough" or "I can't do anything right" or "I don't deserve happiness" are unconsciously imparted to us by our parents, our church, and our culture. Shame and guilt are the cornerstones of these destructive beliefs.

Shame and Guilt

If shame reflects who we think we are, as in "I'm so ashamed of myself," then guilt involves what we do, as in "I feel guilty about what I did." Shame and guilt prohibit us from realizing who we truly are. They also serve as a protection against the experience of painful emotions. They provide a way to avoid taking responsibility for our actions. (It is similar to blame, which is one way we release ourselves from guilt and shame.)

Through our feelings of guilt, we create a subtle form of punishment. The contraction we feel as a result sends us back to repeat the negative behavior we felt guilty about to begin with. This cycle of punishment and expiation is a misuse of our vital energy. When we indulge our guilt, we are saying no to who we are and feeling self-righteous about it at the same time.

Guilt has a lot of justification and righteousness about it. When we fail to listen to the intuition of our healer, and then abuse ourselves, we usually feel guilty about it afterward. We believe that by subjecting ourselves to the discomfort of guilt, we are repenting for our sins. This allows us to repeat our behavior since we have already suffered for it.

Guilt is a way of justifying an undesired behavior pattern. This is actually a very primitive technique. It's as if we were doing penance to the gods, who take pity on our suffering and absolve us of our sins. Unfortunately, this primitive cycle drains our energy, which could be redirected more creatively into choices that support healing.

Shame and Sexuality

By stepping out of this cycle and not falling back into the trap of guilt, we can begin to look at the feelings of shame we are trying so desperately to escape from. For instance, one of my clients who was especially plagued by his repressed homosexuality was willing to do virtually anything to avoid the shame of his sexual preference. He was so afraid of rejection that he lied about his feelings. He pretended that he was someone he was not, while denying who he was.

He became engaged to marry an unsuspecting classmate when he was nineteen, but grew to be resentful of having to hide his true feelings. He would sabotage the relationship by provoking abusive fights with her, then feel guilty about it and beg her to take him back. Finally in therapy he admitted his attraction toward other men and began to say yes to those feelings. In one breakthrough session, he broke down sobbing, releasing years of repressed energy. His ability to finally say yes to who he was created room for healing. He amiably broke off his engagement shortly afterward and embarked on a gradual path of acknowledging his homosexuality to himself, his family, and his friends.

My client's shame was not only reinforced by society; in some ways it was created by it. The covert as well as open violence and discrimination toward gays and other minorities that pollutes our society, encourages victim consciousness in all of us. If we judge another in order to feel superior, then we are prisoners of that judgment ourselves. If we succumb to the judgment from others, somewhere it reflects a self-judgment that we could be still carrying from childhood. Then, as a defense mechanism, we wear the mask of the blamer, and blame society, creating a vicious cycle with no room for understanding.

An example of this is the atmosphere of guilt and shame created by the church and media around the subject of AIDS. Some limited thinkers cruelly suggest that gay men should be ashamed of the fact that they have AIDS, and that they should feel guilty for whatever they did to contract it. This belief is based exclusively on fear, and has absolutely no basis in truth.

If a person with AIDS holds such a belief to be true, it might suggest that somewhere deep within his subconscious he holds a similar shame-based belief. With this awareness, he can begin to release the early childhood programming that says homosexuality is bad and replace it with an affirmation of self-acceptance and self-love.

I have observed this passage with a number of my clients as they move from their identity as AIDS *victim* to become a person with AIDS. But there still are some core beliefs that need to be weeded out to allow them to step out of victim consciousness. These weeds need to be dug out at the roots. Let us consider the issue of punishment.

Punishment

One day in session with a very dear friend and client, I asked him to speak about his feelings concerning punishment. He shared his theory that punishment did not really exist in our universe, and said that he was far beyond operating at that level of conscious-ness. Tuning in to him, I noticed how strong his defensive energy was. Because it felt like I was hitting a wall of concrete, I knew it was too soon to explore the real truth behind his words.

At the next session he arrived quite agitated and admitted that my question concerning punishment had really upset him. He went on to express his surprise and consternation that a spiritually evolved being such as myself was still operating at such a base level of consciousness. He then quickly changed the subject to the dif-ficulty in his relationship, and we focused the session on that issue.

The following session, he brought up the subject of punish-ment again, and said that it was annoying him terribly, and that I was responsible for upsetting him. Very softly I reminded him about his theory that punishment didn't exist and that he had evolved beyond it. He became very angry and was finally able to express his frustration. He confessed that his theory was merely an intellectual concept and that he was unable to live it yet. I asked him to close his eyes and to express his feelings concerning punishment. Expressions of guilt, shame, and punishment were followed by a storm of tears and emotion. After his release, he felt a sense of lightness and liberation.

We cannot push the river of healing. As I keep reminding you, healing is an allowing. Yet we sometimes become impatient and, instead of allowing time for our resistance to dissolve organically and for certain aspects of the condition to resolve, we rush the healing process. This is when we don the mask of the pusher. In fact this survival mask shows up in all areas of our lives, and has often contributed to the breakdown of our body in the first place.

The Pusher

Our society is neurotic in the way it denies us permission to take care of ourselves in our own time. Unless we are faced with a catastrophic condition, we feel we have to continue to live in the fast lane, wearing the mask of the pusher, pretending that "I can handle it" until our body finally can't handle it anymore.

The pusher can really get in the way of healing. For example, there is an aspect of New Age thinking that is a direct result of the pusher. Throughout the past few years, I have heard many clients make statements like, "I have to face my anger" or "I have to get rid of my denial." Usually, when I delved deeper into it, I discovered that the "denial" was a label projected onto my clients by a previous therapist, teacher, or associate.

For instance, I worked with one client who judged himself harshly for not being able to tell his parents or colleagues at work about his AIDS-related condition. He had been participating in HIV-positive support groups that emphasized the importance of "coming out" and owning the condition as a positive step toward healing. This of course is ultimately true, yet if it is forced prematurely, it can result in more harm than good. In the case of my client, he compared himself to the standards of others, and subsequently felt more shame because he wasn't "doing it right."

The Comparer

Comparison is poison and is another way we perpetuate our sense of unworthiness. Comparing our bodies, our clothes, our cars, our lovers, our successes, or even our failures with those of others robs us of the ability to appreciate who we are, where we are on our journey, and what we're doing in our present moment.

We reinforce our sense of shame and unworthiness by comparing ourselves with the pictures and messages we are bombarded with by the media. The standards set by the cultural icons of our day are so impossible to meet that there are very few of us who don't feel inferior in comparison.

Comparing is like a cancer of the heart. It consumes our love, and by continuously making judgments about good and bad, we set up expectations and limit our experience. We lose the possibility of embracing our own uniqueness, and in doing so we cripple our ability to participate consciously in the miracle of life.

Comparing prevents us from experiencing the fullness of the present moment. For example, when I received my diagnosis, I immediately compared how it was before with how it is now, and mourned my tragic loss. I compared my present situation to how life used to be, lamented my shattered dreams, and grieved my stolen health.

At the same time, I felt almost relieved that I no longer had to endure the stress of my old life and the pain of Nado's rejection. Again I compared my present with my past, but this time I rationalized in a distorted way that I was better off sick. I also welcomed the "special attention" I received for being sick.

The Manipulator

As I mentioned earlier, when I was a child I used disease to manipulate those around me, Often it was the only time my mother would give me the special attention I craved so badly. When I first became ill, I thought I was using disease to manipulate Nado, but as I discovered later, the person I was ultimately manipulating through my disease was myself.

In our society with its emphasis on self-reliance and independence, we often feel that under normal circumstances we should not ask for help or support. When we are diagnosed with a life-threatening illness, however, it suddenly is socially acceptable to become dependent on others for the care and compassion we crave and deserve.

Even though care and compassion is our birthright, the inner child in us feels that we don't deserve it unless we are suffering as our way to earn it. Because our inner child equates special attention with love, which equals survival, she will do anything to get it. This includes wearing the mask of the manipulator and using disease as a tool to get love. This distorted attitude feeds and perpetuates the role of disease in our lives and is a form of self-abuse.

The Indulger and Self-abuse

As a collective culture we have lost our inborn sense of trust; as a result, our present society is extremely abusive. Many of us have experienced an emotionally and in some cases physically or sexually abusive childhood, which has created a deep sense of mistrust within us.

Most of the time, in order to realize the full impact of it, we need a very strong wake-up call from the universe. Even then it demands strong discipline and a helpful support system to empower us to disconnect from the habit of self-abuse, and the pattern of abuse to and from others. In a strange way, we become addicted to the intensity of abuse. Often we are not able to recognize the full impact on our physical bodies until it is too late.

For many people with AIDS, self-abusive behavior like repeated anonymous sex or drug abuse generated deep and destructive wounds, although these people were not necessarily aware of it at the time. For example, the search for sex is really a search for love. It is the need to be held, to connect with another human being, yet it is often sabotaged by a greater fear of intimacy and rejection. In the case of a drug abuser, drugs are a way to escape contraction in search of artificial expansion. Many users are seeking the light that they experienced when they first experimented with drugs, when their consciousness first opened up beyond the illusion of "reality."

As a therapist, I see many clients who have used their energy in a very abusive way. Even though some of them now know what steps they need to take to support their healing, they still indulge their child survivor's "needs," believing that the payoff will be worth the abuse. Many of them continued to justify and rationalize their choices to stay in abusive relationships, use drugs, eat poorly, work at a frustrating job, or continue to have anonymous unsafe sex, denying the consequences.

Waking up to heal one's life takes great courage, and there is no way around it, yet the indulger is a master at trying to find the easy way. The indulger is simply another defense mechanism of the child survivor and is a reaction to an old survival program. The indulger is one of the greatest opponents to healing.

When we are operating from indulgence, we are unable to listen to the healer within, who can show us the way to make a different choice. I have observed a drastic positive change in virtually all of my clients when first they are willing to acknowledge the indulger in them, see its impact on their life, and then discontinue their self-abusive behavior.

The self-abusive pattern often continues after they have stopped the behavior due to their feelings of shame and guilt. Before they can utilize the different tools that facilitate the healing process, they need to become aware of the source of these abusive patterns. The mastery of the healer is to recognize that these patterns are there and then be willing to let them go.

Letting go of a self-destructive pattern, such as an addiction or an abusive relationship, takes a lot of courage and self-mastery. It is usually best to completely remove ourselves from the abusive environment first. Being around others who are still indulging in the self-destructive behavior does not support healing, and usually hinders it. Most of the time, it is imperative that we disconnect totally from our old environment. It may seem brutal, but it is a necessary passage. It is vital to create in its place a new "family" or support system with values that support our healing.

The Supportive Clan

Because modern society has lost the sense of clan and family, the deep, traumatic wounds from abusive childhoods tend to remain open and sore. They have no safe place to heal, no time for the scar to form. Today, the clan, with its sense of security and community, is mostly found in twelve-step programs, support groups, spiritual communes, and therapeutic workshops. These groups can support the passage from self-abuse to self-love. In these groups people are willing to receive each other openly, without judgment, so that the repressed emotional energy from those traumatic events can be released and heal.

That is why I continue to emphasize the importance of surrounding yourself with a support system, or a community of people on the same path. Our individual stream can dry out in the desert of the outside world. By connecting with other streams, we can create a river on the way to the ocean. This river becomes a silent conspiracy to transform and heal our planet. In fact, transformation is already happening on many levels as a result of this kind of grassroots conspiracy, which is riding the accelerated wave of personal and planetary evolution.

The child survivor thinks she knows all the answers, all the ways to avoid pain, and uses every trick she can to survive. The child survivor is a wonderful machine designed to protect us from harm, and we can be grateful to her for doing her job. The key is to remember that most of what the child survivor perceives as harm is an imaginary projection from the past onto the present or future.

Very rarely is the child survivor willing to see what is really happening in our life. For example, let's say you tell someone you are attracted to them, and would like to go on a date together, and the other person says that he or she is busy that night. The child survivor may interpret that response as rejection, which would then trigger a whole string of reactions, coming from the child survivor's fear of death if she were to be rejected by her parents.

By slowly and steadily cleansing the filters of our perception through emotional release and meditation, we are able to begin to wake up to what is real, here and now in this moment. Everything else is imaginary. *Everything.* There is only *now* and there is only *here;* everything else is an illusion of the mind.

It is as if we are walking around with photographic slides that represent the memories of our past and the expectations of our future, and we are projecting them onto the people, places, and things in our present reality. Healing evolves when we wake up to the fact that the pictures in our minds are simply memories, which cannot harm us because they no longer exist. They happened yesterday, or last year, or long ago, but they are not happening now.

Because we were not able to completely express our emotions during many of these past events, the memories are like ghosts haunting us in search of completion. Because of these ghosts, we still react to the projection of those memories as if they were happening today, making us blind to the fact that we are contaminating the present with our past. In healing, it is our responsibility to recognize that life always changes, bringing us new opportunities to transcend our old limited ways and open up to a more masterful way of being. Then we are ready to stop trying to survive, and discover what it is to live.

P R O C E S S

Strategies of the Child Survivor

This process examines one of the major strategies of the child survivor: *wanting life to be different.* The child survivor thinks that if she can always get her way, then she will be happy. She will use all of her masks to accomplish that end, including those of the controller, the complainer, and the manipulator.

Unlike the other processes, do *not* read this one all the way through first; instead read each section only as you do it. It is important, whenever you do this process, that you do all four sections in one sitting. This process can be used over and over as a way to understand your child survivor.

1. Open your journal to a blank page on the left-hand side. Write the following question on the top of the page.

> *What can other people do that I can't?*

Make a list of all the answers that are relevant to your life. Your child believes if only you could do or have these things, then you would be happy.

2. When you feel you have answered as many as you can for now, go down the list one by one, filling in the blank with each answer.

> *I don't want to* _____

For example, if the answer is . . . "be in a happy relationship," then you would say out loud: "I don't want to . . . be in a happy relationship."

3. When you have completed the list, start at the beginning again and notice which answers create expansion in you because they resonate as truth. Allow yourself the freedom to let go of those old desires that no longer serve you. Then observe which answers create contraction in you, because of a sense of longing or gnawing from unfulfilled desires. Allow yourself to feel any feelings of anger, frustration, or sadness that may arise.

4. Now on the right-hand page, make a list of answers to the second part of the statement.

I don't want to . . . because if I did _____

For example, "I don't want to . . . be in a happy relationship, because if I was . . . I would have to give up my freedom. (You may change the verb if it is appropriate to correspond to the answer.)

17

Contraction

Just as the seed that starts its life in the darkness of the soil, or the child that starts its life in the darkness of the womb, all beginnings are in the dark because darkness is one of the most essential things for anything to begin. The beginning is mysterious, hence darkness is needed. It is also very intimate, that's also why darkness is needed. Darkness has depth and a tremendous power to nourish.

—OSHO

CONTRACTION is tension. It is an instinctive reaction to pain and discomfort. It is an attempt to control the energy of fear, anger, and sadness, but paradoxically it is also the source of that energy. Contraction stretches across the whole spectrum of darkness, reaching all the way to evil.

Because contraction is analogous with our dark side, it may sound like something purely negative, perhaps even dangerous. Yet it is an essential step before expansion. Just as in the birthing process, where the contractions of the mother push the baby out of the darkness of the womb into the light of day, it is the pain and contraction in our lives that push us to reach our maximum potential.

Contraction is going within. It is part of the natural cycle of the universe and shows us continuously what needs to be examined, what is ready to heal, or what we can let go of in our lives.

It is not something bad that we need to transcend. This is a major misunderstanding on the path of healing.

In our society we refuse to accept the dark side of ourselves, and do everything we can to avoid it. Consequently very few of us take the time to focus inward. Tremendous fear has been generated by our attitude toward darkness. When we resist and deny contraction, we feed it even more. When we suppress it and pretend it does not exist, contraction takes on a disproportionate dimension in our lives.

Left alone, the natural flow between contraction and expansion does not harm us. Yet, when it is disrupted by our minds, which judge it as good or bad or try to direct or control it, it will ultimately destroy us. In order to return to the natural flow between contraction and expansion, we need to accept responsibility for the disharmony that we created through our resistance and control in the first place.

Accepting the Challenge

When we don't resist contraction, it becomes a useful tool for growth and expansion in our daily lives. Contraction serves us by challenging us to be the best we can be. It's like the old farmer whose wheatfields had produced a poor harvest for several years. He blamed it on the difficult elements of nature, and asked God for perfect weather and an end to harmful insects and weeds. The old farmer prayed every day until finally one day God answered his prayers and created a perfect environment exactly as the farmer had requested. No thunderstorms, no weeds, and no bugs. The wheat grew so high that the farmer thanked God for His generosity and abundance.

When the crops were finally harvested there was no wheat inside. The farmer was dumbfounded. He asked God what had gone wrong and God responded that the wheat was empty because there was no struggle, no conflict. Since everything that was considered bad had been avoided, there was no challenge and therefore no reward. It is the obstacles in life that challenge us to reach our maximum potential.

When we accept the challenge and do whatever is necessary in response to it, we usually experience a natural state of expansion afterward, as when we finish a race in spite of our exhausted body, or when we assert ourselves with our boss or our doctor. This natural expansion then creates room for all the contraction we have repressed in our package, all those traumas that never healed, all the demons we keep locked inside, to come to the surface. Instinctively we contract again. We resist and deny. We'll do anything to avoid the pain of our disowned feelings.

It is vitally important to remember that no matter at what point on your journey this repressed energy surfaces, you should say yes to it as part of the healing process. It is so liberating to express anger and sadness. When we accept our feelings, both positive and negative, we open the door for healing to begin. Life, after all, has its moments of happiness and despair, no matter how spiritually evolved we think we are. That's just the way *it* is. If we can acknowledge *it,* and stop resisting *it,* we can be nourished by *it.*

If we insist on seeking only one part of the cycle (as in some schools of spiritual thought which only acknowledge the light), then we create imbalance. Healing exists in the space between the dark and the light, in the dance of contraction and expansion.

For example, many people who work with me feel wonderful in the beginning, and then suddenly as their repressed feelings emerge, they feel terrible and want to stop. But guess what: the healing process is not comfortable. It may hurt for a while to go farther, but once you've moved through the contraction, it won't have such a destructive influence on you.

Those who persevere and accept whatever comes up receive the reward of a fruitful harvest. Those who give up and search for another technique or another teacher are only postponing the weeding process. Those who plant their seeds too close to the surface in an effort to avoid having to dig too deep will find that the roots will not be substantial enough to support the plant's maximum growth.

This process of accepting the bad with the good is especially challenging for people with AIDS. Many of the people I have worked with receive great insight through their daily meditation, only to lose trust in their own power to heal when they next contract an opportunistic infection (as I did when I was first diagnosed). Almost like jilted lovers, they discard their daily meditation, and their intuitive guidance while seeking the magic cure.

This stage of your journey can be a major turning point in your healing process. If you should find yourself sick in bed, faced with the challenge of an opportunistic illness, I invite you to slowly begin to acknowledge your fears and whatever feelings they bring up. It may be anger or frustration or despair. Use the time alone to express whatever you are feeling. (A process on releasing negative emotion is included in the next chapter.)

Allow yourself also to say yes to the part of you who wants to get rid of the disease at any cost—the child survivor, who will do anything to avoid death, including all kinds of meditation, and medication. Don't repress any part of you; let all the feelings come up and out.

It may also serve you to meet the part of you who judges the disease as a threat, another response of your child survivor. He may also judge your healing process as a failure. Allow that to be okay, for now. Instead of wasting precious healing energy trying to change, allow yourself just to be for a while. Let yourself float downstream, until you gain back the strength to actively resume your journey. The long-distance runner knows how to pace herself. The mountain climber knows when to rest.

As we can begin to recognize all the various fragmented parts of ourselves, and not judge one as better than the other, then we can start to see where we are conflicted and where we are aligned. When we can honor all parts of our life, including the illness itself, we immediately experience expansion. It is in that expansion that healing occurs. Once we say yes to the feelings of contraction, the natural flow of the universe carries us back to the cycle of expansion and contraction and we continue the dance between them.

Contraction in our Body

As we begin to accept contraction as half of the natural cycle, and not judge it as a negative state, the next step is to identify our physical responses and where the energy is located in our body. We tend to hold the contraction which relates to negative emotions in specific areas. For instance, many people contract with anger in their hand, throat, forehead, and pelvic area. The hand represents action, the throat expression, the forehead psychic vision (the third eye), and of course the pelvic region corresponds to sexual expression and creativity. Repressed anger in any area of our life could show up as contraction in the corresponding area of our body. Sadness frequently gets held in the center of the chest, while anxiety and fear contract in the stomach, solar plexus, and shoulders. Thus sadness corresponds to the heart center, and anxiety and fear connect with the areas of the body that symbolize power (the solar plexus) and responsibility (as in "I feel like I'm carrying the world on my shoulders").

In a vicious circle, the contraction represses the emotional energy even further and eventually builds up to the point of creating an imbalance and distortion in the body, as seen in hunched shoulders. It can also cause chronic conditions such as ulcers and migraines, and can even lead to serious illnesses such as cancer.

Once we identify contraction, it can be released. But according to our general rule of healing, we can't *do* a release, we have to *allow* it. The first step is to say yes to the contraction as it is. As we explore the contraction and its location in our body, it begins to melt away on its own. Our gentle awareness and acceptance is all that is needed for it to transform. If we try to change or fix it, we risk the possibility of creating more contraction around the contraction, which will keep us stuck in it even longer.

P R O C E S S

A Bioenergetic Exercise
on Contraction

This exercise is effective in releasing repressed energy locked inside
your body. When energy is released, it can be redirected and used
for healing.

Several clients were in such extreme states of contraction when
they first came to work with me that they could barely express
themselves. One of them was so depressed that his doctor had
diagnosed him as chronically depressive and was preparing to admit him to a psychiatric hospital for chemical treatment. When I
tuned in to him I could feel his despair and his resistance to it. Since
he was unable to find an expression for his feelings, he stuffed
them, and labeled himself a failure. Through this exercise he was
able to release the contraction and begin to say yes to the long-
repressed feelings of anger and despair.

I invite you to read the whole process through first, and then
follow the directions. Take out the journal or notebook that you
have chosen as a support tool for your healing journey. Open it
to a clean page and write the word "Contraction" on the top
line.

Let your eyes close and tune in to all the areas of contraction
in your life. For example, your current physical condition, or a
difficult relationship. When you are ready, open your eyes and list
each source of contraction in your journal. Take your time. This
process is private. It is for you only, so you need not hide anything.
When you complete the list, put the journal down in front of you
so that you can read it, and stand up in the center of the room.

Let your eyes close again, and take a few deep breaths. Now
tune in to each item on the list and let yourself feel the sensations
of contraction. If you feel yourself wanting to escape, take another
deep breath and bring yourself deeper into the feeling. Allow your
entire body to feel whatever discomfort there is. Where is it lo-

cated? Your neck, your lower back, your stomach? What does it feel like? Is it a dull ache, a throbbing pain? Is your breathing affected? Your heartbeat?

Now, letting your instincts guide you, allow your body to move in a way that expresses the sensation of contraction. For instance, your muscles may tighten, or your body may feel like it is becoming very small. You may curl into the fetal position, or hide in a dark corner or under a table. Whatever it may be, allow your body to express it.

Once you feel connected with your body's sensation of contraction, take a deep breath, hold it, and go into the contraction even further. If the fear of rejection is what makes you contract, go into the feeling of being rejected and experience it fully as you hold your breath and tighten your body. Face the feeling totally by holding your breath for as long as you can, focusing your entire energy on the experience of rejection (or whatever is the source of your contraction).

When you have gone totally into your contraction and can hold your breath no longer, exhale forcefully, allowing your body to feel the release of energy. Tune in to your body. Is the contraction still present? If so, where? Has it moved or changed?

Choose another source of contraction from your list and allow yourself to go into that feeling totally. Has the contraction disappeared? What are you feeling now? Expansion? Lightness? Emptiness? Take a few deep breaths and allow your breathing to return to normal. Let your eyes open and record your body's responses in your journal. Here is a format you can use:

SOURCE	INTENSITY	LOCATION	CHANGE
rejection	diluted, not easy to connect	my whole body, difficulty breathing	easier to breathe
AIDS diagnosis	extremely strong, like a pounding	my temples, stomach, neck	less intense

Be gentle with yourself when you have completed. Put on some soft music, meditate, or take a bubble bath. Do something to nurture yourself. This process can be done often and does not require the assistance of anyone else. Whenever you feel extremely physically or emotionally tense, this exercise can help you release it.

The Contraction of Fear

When we finally move through our denial and resistance, we usually experience tremendous fear. We become afraid of the overwhelming intensity of our feelings of hopelessness and despair as well as our projected nightmare of the future. When I finally began to face the inescapable reality of my disease after months of denying the symptoms, I discovered that the vulnerable child in me was terrified.

Like denial, resistance, and control, fear is a tool of the child survivor. It is a reaction to such early childhood judgments as "People cannot be trusted" or "The world is not a safe place." Our subconscious reaction of fear happens so instantaneously that it is virtually instinctual.

Fear as Survival Instinct On the most basic level, fear is actually a survival instinct. When we are in danger, all our senses are alert, and our awareness becomes sharpened. While in the state of fear, we are able to evaluate the life-threatening situation and choose the appropriate behavior, either fight or flight. That is the basic purpose of fear, which we all know either consciously or unconsciously. It is a healthy sign that our instinct is functioning well.

The quantum leap that is possible for us at this time in human history is to realize that we have mastered the majority of our actual survival fears; but we are not yet aware of it. Because of our blindness we have created new fears to replace the ones that we have mastered. For example, when mankind lived in caves, exposed and vulnerable to the many forces of nature, including wild

animals, we did not have the tools and weapons to defend ourselves, and we lived in fear. We also lived in fear of other tribes,
because they were our predators and a threat to our survival.

We have mostly mastered those conditions, except for the
weather and certain warring "tribes" who fight amongst themselves over power, land, and religious differences. Basically we have
been able to master all our other sources of fear, in terms of actual
survival. Except in cases of racial, religious, and social discrimination, almost every individual is able to find food and shelter without risking his or her life. (The reason everyone does not have the
same opportunity has more to do with politics, greed, and preju-
dice than with the threat of nature, but that is the subject for
another book in itself.)

Most of us have mastered the real day-to-day survival threats,
or are able to approach agencies to assist us in doing so. Because
these fears are so ingrained in our genes, however, we use our new
awareness and development as a way to protect ourselves against
imaginary survival threats. For instance, many people nowadays
fall into what I call the "New Age trap," using crystals, meditation,
and their higher guides to protect themselves against negativity.
Not only are these people giving their power away, but they are
also perpetuating their same old fear patterns by making the fear
more real. The transformational breakthrough that is available for
us now, as an entire species, is to let go of these ancient fears, to
stop perpetuating them, and to discover who we are when the
energy of fear is transformed.

The Fear of the Child Another kind of fear that comes from our past
conditioning is what I call the fear of the child. It is usually an
anxiety response to an imaginary or exaggerated situation, based
on all of the subconscious programming we are still carrying.

To the child, the prospect of riding in an airplane, swimming
in the ocean, or walking into a room full of strangers can seem
utterly terrifying even if there is no apparent or immediate danger
involved. This sort of anxiety in an adult is actually a reaction to

an early childhood memory that has been reactivated by a thought, feeling, or incident in the present environment. The reaction of fear usually has very little to do with the present, if anything at all. Because the child interprets everything on a literal level, the fear of rejection can be as frightening as the crash of a Boeing 747.

An important step in healing is to acknowledge the fear and to determine whether it is actually justified right now, in this very moment. If it is an actual life-threatening moment, such as a high fever, a mugging, or a car skidding on the road, we can react appropriately and take the proper lifesaving measure. If we determine that the fear is not justified in our present circumstances—that our survival is not being threatened right now—then we can look at what life decisions from our past are generating these fears.

Fear as a Useful Tool Fear can also serve as a useful tool in our daily lives. If we approach our fear with gentle acceptance, it can teach us how to take care of the vulnerable child within, and motivate us to live from a place of integrity. It is not the fear itself that is making us sick, but rather the repressed energy inside of us, especially when we don't believe we have any tools to deal with our fear.

One of my greatest fears, for example, is that I might end up homeless. This comes from my early childhood fear of abandonment. Ironically, since I became a spiritual disciple, and because I travel so much leading workshops, I have learned to release my child's attachment to the "security" of owning a big home filled with beautiful possessions. Because my child's fear of being homeless sometimes returns strongly, one of the logical ways I take care of her, is by making a commitment to pay my rent on time!

Say Hello to Fear When we let our fears run our lives we become single-mindedly obsessed with how to avoid or get rid of what we fear. Paradoxically, there is nothing we can do to directly dismiss or get rid of fear. The more we try to conquer it, the stronger it becomes. The problem is that the moment fear arises, it creates dual personalities—one who has the fear, and one who wants to get rid of it. This duality creates confusion and conflict, and sabotages the healing process.

The way to transcend fear is by first embracing it. Say hello to the terrified young one inside of you, without trying to change him or her. Become interested in what some of these conscious and subconscious fears are, and what decisions they are based on. For instance, I have been afraid of the dark since I was very young. My fear is still there. It hasn't changed. When I am in the dark, I get scared, but then I use my awareness to realize "Oh, it's you again, my old fear of the dark. This is who I am in this moment." This is the way we heal our fear, by recognizing it, taking a deep breath, and saying hello.

Recently I have been dealing with another one of my fears, the fear of putting my head underwater. I love the ocean, as you know, but because I nearly drowned fifteen years ago, putting my head underwater terrifies me. Because I was planning to swim with the dolphins in the Florida Keys, I wanted to learn how to be comfortable swimming underwater again.

One day in Key West, as I slowly entered the ocean, I decided to try to submerge my head underwater just for a moment. At first I was fine, but I reached a point where I couldn't go any farther. I was at a crossroads and I had a choice. I could allow the judge in me to call myself a cowardly wimp, and then allow the pusher in me to force me to put my head underwater again. I could rape myself one more time, and totally negate my child's panic in an effort to "transcend my fear." I could make that choice, and push myself to "heal," but I would have to deal with my child's emotional rape later on. This may seem like an extreme statement, but look for yourself: it's what we do. We expect our frightened child to repress his or her feelings and do what the judge, the controller, and the pusher expect us to do.

The other option was to acknowledge that this was as far as I could go right now, and say hello to that part of me. As I moved through the warm gentle waves, my body was showing me who I was at that moment. I became a "witness" and simply observed what was happening. I could hardly breathe, my knees were weak, my hands were shaking, and I just said hello to all of it.

Several weeks later, while I was swimming with those gentle loving dolphins, I found that the time was ripe to let go of my fear. Because I was totally in the present moment with the dolphins, my mind did not judge the situation as frightening. As I swam in the now, moment by moment, I released the old decision I had made following my near drowning experience. Occasionally when the surf is rough, my fear resurfaces, but when the ocean is gentle, I enjoy the freedom to swim in my beloved ocean.

We are often impatient on our healing journey because the clock is ticking, but healing takes incredible patience. Keep saying hello. "This is where I am today. Maybe tomorrow I will be able to move into deeper water, submerge my face longer. And maybe not."

This is what I call loving myself, and it doesn't fit the picture of the judge or the pusher. Because she wants so desperately to belong, the pusher always forced me to overcome my fears, with no respect for my personal boundaries. She would justify this with all kinds of rationales, such as "You have done so much work on yourself, this should not be an issue. You should be able to dive into the water head-first."

Until we are willing to say hello to our fear and accept it, we can live only at a very superficial level. Part of accepting our fears is knowing that we will continue to experience these unwanted emotions. We don't just heal our fear once and for all. It continues to come and go, like the tide. Each time it rises, if we say yes to it, we can move through it. For centuries, Western man has tried to escape his fears or conquer them by force. This is the male, aggressive way. It is a *doing*. My invitation to you is to begin to approach the healing of your fears in the feminine, receptive way, which is an *allowing*, a letting go.

The Influence of Fear As I mentioned earlier, our governments and religions have manipulated the masses through fear for generations. Army training represents an extreme example of an attitude which permeates our society on all levels. Soldiers are manipulated through fear to become perfect killer machines. Yet I believe that if I were to sit with them individually for a few hours, until they felt safe enough to open up and share their true feelings, the majority of them would admit that they really don't want to kill anyone.

Because our society is ruled by fear, the child within will do everything he can to be "good," including denying that he is afraid. Living with repressed anxiety, always ready for fight or flight, takes an undue toll on our bodies and minds. Our life force, which supports our immune system, is continually being drained by the stress of living in a constant state of emergency.

When we are dealing with a life-threatening illness our fears can become even more intensified because we are finally face-to-face with the fear behind all fears: death. It has always been there, lurking in the shadows, but we never dealt with the reality of it.

When I was first diagnosed with ARC, I was consumed with fear for my children, for Nado, and for myself. As a result my symptoms worsened rapidly. I was constantly examining my body for progressive symptoms as a way to validate my fear of the nightmare that lay ahead. This of course only made both my fear and my symptoms worse. It wasn't until I finally embraced my fears and surrendered to my inevitable death that the symptoms began to mitigate.

When we live in fear, there is no room for joy, for passion, for stillness, for being. We always need to do something as a way to protect ourselves: earn more money, acquire more knowledge, build a better body, take more drugs, in some cases even buy a gun. Whatever the survival tool is, our lives become ways to escape and avoid fear.

On the healing journey, it is very important to learn to embrace our fears and release them. Remember that most of our fears are not real. They are based on old memories that cannot harm us. It's as if we are believing the old movies in our minds and projecting them on our present lives.

P R O C E S S

Fear as a Useful Tool

This process will help you to face your fears, embrace them, and then release them. Do *not* read it through entirely, but read it as you go along, step by step.

1. First sit in a comfortable chair and take a few deep breaths. Close your eyes and allow yourself to remember the fears that are most frightening to you.

2. Open your eyes, and list all of your fears in your journal. Include the chronic fears from your childhood, as well as those fears that are currently plaguing your life. Place a check mark next to those fears that are most alive in you, and that carry the most energy.

3. One by one go down the list and say the following affirmations in a strong, clear voice, filling in the blanks with each fear you selected.

I recognize that the fear of _____ *is a useful tool and I accept it.*

[Inhale and exhale deeply.]

I now release the energy of fear of _____ .

[Inhale and exhale deeply.]

I now allow healing energy to replace fear energy.

Rest for a minute between each fear, allowing yourself to feel the healing energy replacing the fear energy. Then continue with the next fear until you have completed the list.

The Contraction of Anger

During those times when the fear became too overwhelming I used anger as a way of coping with the tremendous terror my child was feeling. At first I was unable to express my rage. I played the victim role, accusing and blaming everything and everyone around me. Eventually I said yes to my anger, and allowed the repressed energy to move. It was partly by releasing my anger in a healthy, nonviolent way that I was able to create the empty space for healing.

What is anger, anyway? Most of the time we define anger by our reaction to it. Ask people about their anger and they will tell you how afraid they are of it, how much they try to control it, how they will do anything in order to avoid it—but they are unable to define what it is. Anger creates such strong reactions in us that we repress it with constant judgments.

Anger is simply life force energy moving at a more intense pace.

Anger as a Useful Tool Anger is part of our energy of resistance. It is the result of nonacceptance of the circumstances of our life. Anger is also a way of discovering and maintaining our boundaries. It is a way to communicate what lines should not be crossed, and to protect us from being violated or intruded upon. Anger is warm and passionate. When we don't express our anger, it distorts into violence, which is cold and destructive. Anger is often confused with violence.

Anger is often a reaction to our feelings of frustration and powerlessness, yet it can also be an important defense mechanism. Anger can serve as a defense against pain and against attack. In fact, it can be considered a healthy reflex. If ever we or our loved ones are actually in physical danger and there is no opportunity for flight, then anger and rage can assist us in fighting off the source of attack, or in accessing the strength to deal with the crisis.

Anger is an important tool for survival for many PWAs. Activist programs like ACT UP (AIDS Coalition to Unleash Power) is a positive way for them to direct their rage against the government and the pharmaceutical industry. Channeling anger into community projects and legislative lobbying serves not only their own personal healing but the community at large as well.

Source of Anger Many of us repress our feelings, especially the "bad" ones such as anger, in order to pretend that we are farther "evolved" than we really are. We often redirect our anger and try to change the circumstances as a way to avoid looking at the source of our reaction, and at what buttons are being pushed inside of us. When we are willing to "own" our anger we can then honestly explore what subconscious program our child is responding to and what masks she is wearing. With this awareness we can engage in dialogue with our child and begin to heal the emotional disharmony which contributes to illness in the physical body.

Repressed Anger When we repress our anger, we never face the source of it, and the wound never has the opportunity to heal. In fact, the opposite usually happens: we grow more resentful, which feeds the anger. Because the feeling can be overwhelming and frightening, we continue to repress it.

It may seem as if we have no control over it, and in a way we don't. If rage has been repressed for an extended period of time, then when it finally erupts on its own, it does so as uncontrollable violence. The violence in our society today, when gangs of youth rape and rampage in our parks, parents abuse and murder their children, and mass murderers spew bullets into crowds of people, is a terrifying illustration of what repressed rage can lead to.

Healing requires that we release repressed anger, but before we can do that we need to say hello to it. As we become interested in our own inner process, we can become familiar with what incidents in our lives trigger our anger and what the energy response feels like in our body.

Most of us are running around with neat little packages of suppressed anger inside of us. In our society, especially the areas controlled by religion, much of our anger, sexuality, and even creativity and spontaneity has been repressed. As children we were not always allowed to express our anger naturally. Most of the time we were punished or told to shut up.

As a parent myself, there were times when I judged my children for getting angry. Because my inner child was not comfortable with their free expression of anger, she wore the mask of the authority figure and forbade them from screaming in "my house." As a result, they didn't have an opportunity to allow the anger to flush out of their system.

Say Yes to Anger The key to releasing anger is simply to say yes to our feelings and to create a safe space for our anger to flow. Anger is a part of the natural cycle of contraction and expansion. It comes and goes, yet when it is repressed it gets stuck and becomes dangerous. It can literally create ulcers and tumors.

When we say yes to our repressed energy in a safe environment, such as a workshop or therapy session, we can flush it out, releasing the steam from our "pressure cooker." When we give ourselves permission to experience our feelings of anger—by screaming intensely into a pillow, stamping our feet, or punching a cushion—we free ourselves to move naturally into our next moment.

When we allow anger to flow through us, it will usually transform on its own into the emotion behind the anger. This is usually the feeling we are attempting to avoid. For instance, if we are angry and we allow ourselves to scream, tears of sadness will often follow. The sadness may then be followed by another round of anger or laughter or finally a deep sense of inner peace. This process does not involve lashing out at someone else. It is a very private process.

The Killer In the workshops I facilitate, I use a meditation called Dynamic, designed by Osho. In it participants are invited to bring about a cathartic release of all of their repressed emotional energy. In the beginning it is important that the meditation be properly supervised, because as participants finally express their rage, it often moves into violence and the killer part of them surfaces. The killer within us is designed to protect us against attack. For instance, a mother in danger will instinctively access the rage of the killer as a way to protect her child.

I always knew that there was a killer inside of me, and it terrified me. My controller had always feared reaching that place.

She was afraid that if I released all the emotion I had repressed all these years I would lose control and my dark side would take over. Many of us are afraid we would actually kill or incite others to kill us if we were to express our inner rage totally. We are afraid we would not be able to stop the explosion of suppressed emotions, so we put a lid on our Pandora's box.

There is a killer in each of us. But remember that it is really just powerful energy. It is not intrinsically evil, but it can be destructive if it is disowned. The more we repress the killer, the more dangerous it becomes. Its suppressed force may even burst out of its pressure cooker one day as violence against ourselves or others.

This is why I encourage exploring the killer part of our personality if it shows up at any point on our journey (as I did when I tore Nado's denim jeans into little bits with my bare hands). As we begin to say yes to the killer inside, under the safe supervision of a trained facilitator, it is no longer so frightening. In owning this part of us that we have disowned for so long, we begin to take real responsibility for ourselves, in both thought and action.

So in the healing journey, don't be surprised if you find yourself in a furious rage sometimes. Watch how alive and juicy you are in those moments. Notice how present and how full of energy you are. When you feel anger, there is really no need to direct it at other people, even though the inner child might want to. A pillow can replace anyone, or any situation.

PROCESS

Releasing Anger

(Read through the entire process before doing it.)

By recognizing that anger is simply energy moving at a more intense pace, and that the repression of it can make us sick or even kill us (through violence and abuse), I invite you to use this process to experience the healthy flush that expressing anger can provide.

As children we were taught proper physical hygiene, but we

have never learned how to regularly cleanse ourselves on the emotional level. When we are willing to flush ourselves of all our negative thoughts, literally purging our emotions, we create a still emptiness within. It is in this emptiness that we can hear the quiet, intuitive voice of our inner healer.

As in the other processes, it is important that you create a safe, private space, where you will not be disturbed. It is imperative that you do this process alone. This is because we like to blame others for our misery and release our anger on them. This kind of release is very destructive, and it will feed the anger instead of flushing it out of you. When we direct anger at someone, it is not healing, it is simply the child survivor getting revenge.

Whenever you feel as if you have reached your breaking point, and that you would like to lash out at someone, go to the privacy of your bedroom. Begin to breathe deeply and quickly. Feel all those negative emotions begin to boil inside of you. When you are really in touch with your anger, let yourself go in a temper tantrum. Stamp your feet, make a fist, and begin to beat your bed, or a cushion. Close your eyes so that you can go beyond being self-conscious and return to the source of the anger. (You may look ridiculous, but so what? Nobody is there to see you.) You may want to scream into your pillow, "No!" or "Fuck you!" to whomever or whatever triggered your anger.

After the first release of strong energy, breathe deeply and wait for the second wave of anger to come. This is a crucial point. Anger comes in several waves, each from a deeper and deeper place in us. If you stop after the first flush, only the surface anger will be released. Continue to breathe quickly and intensely. Give yourself permission to be totally alive in it. It might feel very different, because we have been taught to repress it. Now is your opportunity to express it in a safe and clean way so that it will not stew inside of you trying to find a way out. Eventually it will have to be released, either via physical symptoms (skin boils, tumors), or in an emotional outburst all over some innocent bystander.

Allow that second wave to come and beat your bed or scream into a pillow again. When you have finished emptying yourself of the anger you were feeling, another deeper emotion may surface. Sadness. If you find yourself sobbing uncontrollably, do not try to control or stop it. Simply let yourself release the waves of repressed feelings.

When the storm of emotions has finally passed for the moment, a serene quiet will be available. This is the time to let your creativity flow, because it will tend to happen organically. You will be free of whatever negative emotions were plaguing you before, and positive feelings will be available. Allow yourself to look at your life and circumstances from that new, positive attitude. Finish the process with a moment of gratitude toward yourself and your ability to take care of yourself.

18

Expansion

*Silence is all around you. If it enters your
heart, that is more than any answer.*

—OSHO,

The Mystic Rose

EXPANSION IS AN OPEN, feminine, yin way to use our energy,
and contraction is a closed, masculine, yang way to use it. Because
our world has been mostly ruled by one type of energy—the logical, masculine energy—it is out of balance. Therefore it is important to develop the intuitive, feminine part of us so that we may
create a harmony between the two energies. As I have said many
times, healing comes about as a result of the balanced harmony
between contraction and expansion.

In our society, we know a lot about contraction, and how to
survive using the coping strategies of our minds. Yet we know very
little about expansion and how to simply live in our hearts. We
confuse expansion with the superficial satisfaction of the child survivor's "needs" and desires. We equate it with a certain sense of
security, stemming from personal achievement, material success, or
a comfortable lifestyle. Expansion has become synonymous with
the "good life."

True expansion has nothing to do with that. True expansion is
a state of extreme openness, when we are powerfully alert and
utterly vulnerable. True expansion flows from an open heart, when
we are willing to say yes to life as it is.

Most of the time we stumble onto expansion by accident when
we least expect it. The paradox is that we have to do everything we

can to prepare a climate for that "accident" to happen. Meditation, acceptance of what is, and letting go of our addictions (which are artificial sources of expansion) are tools to prepare the foundation.

Letting Go into Expansion

Expansion is a lightness of being that happens when we are willing to stay open and simply witness our thoughts and survival programming without becoming engaged in them. When we accept who we are in each moment without judgment, a new energy organically emerges. It has the quality of strength, vulnerability, wisdom, and compassion. It is no better or worse than contraction, even though many of us judge it as such.

We sustain our connection to expansion not by trying to possess it but by letting it go, and allowing ourselves to move between the natural rhythm of contraction and expansion. Many clients I have worked with have become frustrated with themselves, because of their inability to remain in expansion forever. Unfortunately, they sometimes give up and withdraw from their healing support systems because of their misunderstanding of the harmony of this process.

When we are attached to expansion it creates an impossible expectation of holding onto it. Life is not a pure state of either contraction or expansion but a constant balance of one state with the other. The more we say yes to our feelings of contraction, allowing ourselves to scream or cry, for example, the more we can experience the gentle emptiness of expansion afterward. The awareness of this natural balance of opposites and the continuous cycle of ups and downs creates an open door for a moment of pure beingness, beyond time, beyond fear, and beyond disease.

The Valley of Expansion The still, quiet emptiness that we feel after a great release of energy is expansion in its most natural form. A common example of this kind of expansion that most of us can relate to happens after sex. During sex, both contraction and expansion rise inside of us. At first it is more contraction than expansion, as momentum builds to reach its peak, which for the majority of us is the orgasm. In that total release, we disappear for a moment. We merge into the experience, and the experiencer and the experience become one. In that merging, "we" don't exist as a separate identity. Release takes over and we lose ourselves in the orgasm.

In our society, we worship that moment of "expansion" and we become attached to it because it feels good. We may roll over and fall asleep, or we may want more, building up the energy within us for another great explosion. Either way, we totally miss the real experience. The orgasm is not the expansion, it is just the passage.

Expansion is the valley after the orgasm. It is in the valley that the mystery exists. This is where we rediscover our world, and ourselves, which emerge organically out of us into the light of day. In our society, the valley is not considered part of the experience. The mind comes in and judges that the experience is finished. We may decide to do it again in order to reach the peak again, or move on to something else, but we totally miss the experience of the valley. Expansion lies in the valley, in the beauty, the magic, and the fragility of it.

The valley is a place of surrender. This is why the majority of us are terrified of it, and would rather separate and fall asleep. Yet it is in this valley of expansion that our greatest awareness exists. It is where forgiveness is experienced, where self-love is total, and where the experience of perfection is available. When we are in expansion, our natural inclination to celebrate life comes back effortlessly, and this becomes a doorway to divine expansion or what the masters call bliss. This is when the energies of our mind, body, and spirit are aligned.

Divine Expansion We usually experience our first taste of divine expansion after some kind of uncomfortable or even life-threatening contraction. It shocks us so deeply that it cracks us open to another dimension of life that we were usually not aware existed. That crack can never be closed again. It can be ignored, but once we have had a glimpse, our life will never be quite the same.

When we have had a taste of the divine, two journeys become available. The first one is the journey inward through meditation in which we travel deeper into our inner world and discover the divine being that we truly are. The other is the journey outward. It emerges naturally as a result of the overflow of divine energy from our true essence.

This is actually the secret of holding onto expansion. When we give to others from the overflow of bliss in our hearts, we make it possible for expansion to occur again. It is like breathing—receiving is like the expansion of inhaling, and giving is like the contraction of exhaling. It is a circular flow of energy.

The Courage to Wake Up In a way, there is also a direct parallel between the crescendo of energy before we reach a sexual orgasm, and the crescendo of energy before we reach the moment that I call a wake-up call. It is rarely comfortable, because it usually arrives as a result of contraction and is always an explosion of the past.

When we have a disease, it is impossible to resist the explosion for very long. After the explosion, when we finally embrace the news of our diagnosis, the valley of expansion is available with a fresh perspective never seen before. We can either roll over and go to sleep, or we can stay awake and explore what is available in the mystery of the moment.

Many of us prefer falling asleep and returning to the dreams of the past, oblivious to the fact that the past no longer exists. Just as when we turn our back on our partner as a way to escape the intimacy of the moment following orgasm, we escape intimacy with life.

In the beginning, the principle of expansion demands the courage to wake up and transcend the conditioning of our child survivor. It takes the willingness to explore what it is to live with integrity instead of indulgence, with honesty instead of pretense. It also requires great courage because it is a state of great aloneness.

The valley of expansion is very fragile, because it is so totally new and different. That is why solitude is an important tool for the inner journey, because we often destroy the newness of the experience by talking about it with others. We fruitlessly try to define it by comparing it with the past, yet it is a brand-new experience which has nothing to do with the past. In this new experience we are the new man, and the new woman. We are our true essence, the one who we have been waiting to discover.

Remember, we cannot make expansion happen. We can only make ourselves available to it by being willing to ride the crescendo of life and to take the passage into the valley, even if it is by way of an explosion that shatters our dreams. Sometimes we need to experience a loss to discover the new. If we are attached to what has gone, we invite pain and suffering like a clinging shackle on our ankle, prohibiting our freedom and burdening our journey.

A Gentle Flowering of Humanity When expansion blossoms, naturally on its own, like a flower that we have planted, watered, and weeded, we get drunk on its nectar. All it takes is just one drop, and we get drunk on the divine. This divine expansion, this bliss, is so powerful that it is life-transforming.

In this state of expansion, we become aware of how gentle and sensitive human beings truly are. We are touched by how beautiful and fragile we are, like rare and exquisite flowers. We also discover that, like the petals of a flower, we are not that different from one another.

Expansion is an opportunity to experience the reality of being human, including the suffering and the glory. It is what we have come to this earth to experience. Expansion is also an opportunity to discover what it is to be divine, in a simple and ordinary way. It is an opportunity to experience the peace and harmony of the valley of acceptance until we gather enough energy for a new explosion. Thus we continue our dance of contraction and expansion as life goes on and on and on . . .

Bioenergetic Exercise on Expansion

Try this exercise. Close your eyes for a moment and think about what makes you feel good. For example, what relationships, what music, what pastimes do you value and celebrate? Once you have connected with a thought or an image, start feeling how your physical body responds. Now, travel deeper and observe how you feel emotionally in connection with those thoughts. Maybe you feel lighter and life seems brighter, or maybe you are curious about what today will bring you. You may even find the time to connect with yourself in a gentle, intimate way for a few nourishing moments. Close your eyes and try it.

How was it for you? What was your experience of your own energy? Take a moment to write down some of your observations in your journal.

SOURCE	INTENSITY	LOCATION	EMOTION
a child's smile	easy, warm	the center of my chest	joy
my lover	strong, passionate	all over my body	gratitude, love

Just by being willing to connect with the love within us, we are nourished. We are then able to overflow and to move through life giving of ourselves. Soon we discover that the more we give the more we receive, and the more we overflow the more energy we have. It is a circle of energy which continues replenishing itself, until it is time to go in again and connect with the next level available to us in our growth.

Opening to Self-Love

On the healing journey it is important to acknowledge that we are so crippled by the way we grow up, that we have an immense craving to be loved, while at the same time we are scared to death of it. This is partly because we remember the painful process of losing our connection to our soul child and the source of all love.

Even though we are longing for love, deep down we are terrified of it because at a subconscious level we believe that love equals pain. In fact, we keep collecting evidence to prove that this is true.

In order to return to a state of unconditional love, we have to open the door to our hearts, which was locked shut when we were forced to disconnect from the love of our soul. The passage back to self-love requires the willingness to melt the chains that bind our hearts with the tears of our pain and loss. As our heart opens, all of our repressed, hurt feelings bubble up to the surface to be released and healed. Although this process may be painful while it is happening, it will eventually pass. Finally, feeling our feelings is the key to the opening of our imprisoned hearts. It is the way we can heal the deep wound that closing down our hearts has created in us.

Putting Yourself on the Top of the List At the beginning of my journey, I was very timidly willing to discover how much I loved myself. I needed to constantly remind myself to keep putting myself on the top of the list. For that I needed to be "selfish," not in the sense of putting myself above others, but in terms of generating a new way to approach my life. In doing so, I had to risk being judged and rejected by others. Despite this, I shared my truth, and what my needs were, regardless of whether they would be accepted or not.

Putting yourself on the top of the list may be a challenge for some of you, because many of us have learned that in order to love others we have to put their needs before ours. Although this may not be taught overtly, it is subtly implied in much of our cultural and religious upbringing. For example, I was raised as a Catholic, in a tradition based on suffering and repression where martyrs are canonized as saints. Ironically, I discovered along my healing journey that the more I put myself down the less available I was to truly love another. When I shifted my focus from "out there" to within myself, the golden rule "Love thy neighbor as thyself," resonated from a brand-new perspective. Suddenly the quality of my self-love was a direct reflection of my ability to love others. By putting myself on the top of the list and giving up trying to please everyone, I was serving not only myself but everyone around me.

How Do I Love Myself? The conditional love that we received as infants is a major source of our lack of self-love. At some point on their healing journey, my clients usually ask the question "How do I love myself?" My answer is always the same. I tell them that I do not know how to teach them *how* to love themselves, but maybe it is time that they begin exploring *why* they don't love themselves. When we can understand why, then we can make whatever changes are necessary, and the how will happen organically.

PROCESS

Exploring Self-Love

(Read the entire process first before doing it.)

Create a safe, quiet, and private environment for yourself where you will not be disturbed for at least forty-five minutes. Sit on the floor, your bed, or on a chair facing another chair, with your pillow in front of you. Place your journal and a pen near you in case you want to make any notes at the end of the exercise.

Take a deep breath, with your eyes open, and let yourself disconnect from the energy and pace of your day. Let yourself slow down and become aware of your body sitting in the room. Feel the connection of your body with the mattress, chair, or floor. Let your mind slow down. Ask the following question out loud: "Why don't I love myself?" While asking the question, you are still your present adult, listening to the sound of your voice, and your eyes are still open, connecting you with the reality of this present moment.

Now shift your body and sit on the pillow in front of you. Close your eyes. Let your body take the position that feels the safest and let yourself receive the question "Why don't I love myself?" Let the young voice of the past emerge. Let the series of adjectives and definitions that have followed you since early childhood speak. Let the criticisms and comments that still have a painful impact on your self-confidence have a voice. Allow your subconscious to recall and release each painful memory one by one, as well as whatever emotions are connected with them.

As the unloved child begins to answer, her body might contract into a fetal position. The voice that responds may sound extremely young and say something like, "Mommy told me I was very bad when I did not want to share my toy with my baby brother." "Daddy sighed in disapproval when he looked at my report card." Or "My teacher told me I was slow," "My older sister told me I was ugly," etc. . . . .

As the memories begin to surface, allow yourself to observe and release the feelings connected with them. Perhaps you will feel angry, and this may be followed by a deep sadness. You may find yourself sobbing at the lack of care and concern in the people who originally made those critical comments.

The more you let yourself release those old memories, letting the emotions flood out of you, the clearer you will be afterward. When you feel complete for now, open your eyes and return to the original position in your present reality. Take a deep breath and allow yourself to see how inaccurate those comments are, those judgments that you chose to embody when you were very young.

Take a few more deep breaths and let the emotions settle down, if they have not already settled. Now notice how often the judge in you criticizes you in the same way. "Why are you not able to do this? Why are you afraid of that?" Become aware of how well you have learned and embodied that tone of self-judgment. Notice how you beat yourself up for every little thing that does not meet with your approval. Perhaps now you pretend you are perfect, praising yourself endlessly to others as a way to mask your personal self-hatred.

It is always important to finish the process as the present adult, perhaps embracing the pillow that represents your younger self, in a moment of deep appreciation for the exploration you have just accomplished. Write down any insights or conclusions you have reached about your decisions regarding self-love in your journal.

Standing Up for Ourselves

We have all been conditioned to one degree or another to expect and even revere suffering. We have learned very little about loving ourselves. Therefore standing up for ourselves from self-love takes tremendous courage. Often, the moment we do, the majority will try to cut us down. The role of the priest and the politician is to make our natural inclinations, like personal pride and joy, into sins. This is a very old tactic to control the masses, and has succeeded down through the ages.

The moment we get in touch with our own self-love, we become invincible. The priest and the politician no longer have power over us, because we no longer need approval from others. We confuse approval with love, and misconstrue personal success with self-love. This is why so many of us are searching for love through material success.

Self-love is totally different. It is a kind of self-realization that has nothing to do with material power. It is a state of divine overflowing, where only sharing exists. It is beyond greed and its lack of trust. It does not coldly separate or divide, but merges in a warm unity. It is a natural state of being. It is our birthright, and who else will claim it for yourself besides you? Are you willing to claim it?

By asking this question of your inner child, you can uncover all the decisions that you made as a young child about not loving yourself, and not putting yourself on the top of the list. Focus the light of awareness within yourself, and begin to realize that there is no validity in the comments and criticisms that were imposed on you as a child. They were from people who were responding from the coldness of their conditioning, instead of from the warmth of their hearts.

I recommend that you have this dialogue with your inner child on a regular basis, at least twice a week. Slowly you will begin to discover how invalid it really is not to love yourself, while at the same time you may also discover how comfortable you have become with it. Our inability to love ourselves is so culturally accepted that we are easily able to justify why we don't love ourselves with a myriad of excuses.

The Art of Loving Ourselves The art of loving ourselves is very new, and therefore very little can be said about it. The first step to loving ourselves is to embrace the simple yet magnificent beings that we are. When we learn to accept all of who we are, the good with the bad, and learn to say yes to our life as it unfolds, we can then become a partner of life.

You may ask, If it is that simple, why is it still so difficult? Loving ourselves takes courage. It is being willing to stand up against the collective unconscious, which believes in the original sin of shame. All you have to do is watch the news to grasp how much we all suffer from collective shame. The majority of a news program focuses on the negative side of an event. Tragedy is somehow considered "good" news. A profitable scoop.

Rarely do we see a story about one person caring for another, or the simple but magnificent acknowledgment of a mother taking care of seven children, day after day. The inspiring example of a father sacrificing his personal freedom to earn a living to provide for his family is not considered noteworthy. The acknowledgment of a student succeeding after long hours of studying, in spite of her insecurity, is preempted by the drama of a rape or murder victim. But it is time that both stories be highlighted.

In our society, daily miracles are totally taken for granted, except perhaps by advertising companies, which use these accomplishments (and our longing for acknowledgment for these accomplishments) to sell products.

The Journey from Our Head to Our Heart Imagine what the world would be like if we were willing to be inspired by our lives instead of being discouraged by them. It could be a very different place if we took the time to acknowledge and celebrate ourselves simply for the miracle of being alive. But are you willing? The world can only be transformed if each of us is willing to learn to love ourselves, embracing the awkwardness of the transformation, and then share that love with those around us.

Healing is the willingness to take the journey from our head to our heart. It may be only a short distance, but the journey can take a lifetime. Healing occurs when we live in the expansion of our hearts.

Expansion through Gratitude

Love is the supreme healing energy. When we experience unconditional love, all is perfect, all is aligned, and disease and death are accepted as a part of life.

One of the greatest tools I have discovered for tapping into love is gratitude. When I take the time to be grateful for the magnificent gift of life as it has been presented to me, I don't waste it. When I don't take life force for granted, and appreciate it as the fragile and powerful energy that it is, I assume full responsibility to channel it, to celebrate it, and to share it fully.

The more we let ourselves fall into the energy of gratitude, accepting all of life, the negative with the positive, the more we will receive in all areas of our lives. It is through gratefulness that healing is available. Life then becomes miraculous, as we allow ourselves to live in communion with God, with the light and dark, with all that is.

Gratefulness Process

I invite you to take a few minutes every night before you go to sleep to ask yourself the simple question:

What about today am I grateful for?

Keep asking and answering the question over and over, as you look at all the areas of your life you feel thankful for. Gratitude is a way of recognizing the precious gift that life is and staying open to receive what life has to offer.

The Mind: Servant or Master?

Because healing intrinsically embraces everything as already perfect, or perfectly imperfect, it is important that you do not fall into the trap of judging the mind or the child survivor as an "enemy" or an obstacle of healing that needs to be transcended. This misconception can create unnecessary obstacles and frustration. The mind is a part of us. It is the magical mechanism that makes a wonderful servant but a terrible master. The mind can serve as a tool to observe, understand, and communicate; it is our choice how to use it. We can allow it either to limit or to empower our healing journey.

The Energy of the Soul Most spiritual teachings tell us that the road to enlightenment is through the totally detached awareness of the mind, whereby we simply witness existence itself. This prepares the way for the miracle of falling into the finer vibration of the soul.

To fall into the energy of the soul does not require a teacher, a specific technique, or a miracle; it is always present. Yet it does demand our total participation. It also requires a moment of stillness. There is no way around it. In order to quiet the mind, we must first slow down our whole life, moving from the survival mode of doing, back to the soul energy of being. This takes tremendous discipline. Meditation is the simplest way I know to quiet down the body with all of its reactions. Then the mind can organically slow down as well, and the passage to reconnect with the soul becomes more available.

Meditation

In meditation, we are constantly meeting our various survival masks, thoughts, and beliefs. As an enlightened master once said, meditation is the willingness to experience one insult after another: the insults of the mind. For example, "I should this, I shouldn't that. Am I doing it right?" Meditation is a magical place to meet the personality of the child survivor, and the endless chatting that constantly takes us away from the present moment.

When I speak of meditation, I am not referring to guided imagery, visualization, or deep relaxation, which serve the purpose of giving the child survivor a sense of relief or a moment of comfort. The meditation that I am referring to is the inner journey of self-discovery. It includes meeting the child survivor, with all of her survival masks, as well as the soul child and the healer.

In meditation we become a witness and simply watch our thoughts, emotions, and physical sensations without judgment. We don't become engaged in our thoughts; we observe them. If we judge, we simply observe that we are judging. Nothing to do. Just watch with gentle detachment. Like white clouds floating effortlessly against a clear blue sky. Meditation is a way to say hello to the chatter of our mind, instead of trying to transcend it or get rid of it. Meditation is a way to discover who we are not, which is one of the first steps in discovering who we are.

Meditation is a doorway to the healer within, because the healer can be accessed only through the acceptance of each moment as it unfolds. This is because the healer is of a very different quality than the child survivor. The healer is expansive, vulnerable, and allowing, as compared to the child survivor, who is contracted, resistant, and controlling.

When we let ourselves fall into the simple and clear energy of the healer, we accept where we are on our journey and recognize that we are still living in a stage of purification. As we flush out our repressed emotions, our mistaken perceptions, and the limited conditioning of the child survivor, we prepare for our reawakening to the magnificent souls that we are.

P R O C E S S

Nadabrahma Meditation

(Read the entire process first before doing it.)

The Nadabrahma meditation, which was designed by Osho, is an important tool in my healing work. It is the meditation that I did every day during my healing journey. I chose Nadabrahma as my daily meditation because the other active meditations were too strenuous for my body at the time. As it turned out, the meditation not only served me on a mental and spiritual level, but on a physical level as well.

Nadabrahma is based on an old Tibetan technique of humming through the nose, and it seems that the humming vibration has a twofold effect. First it helps to focus your energy inwardly, and to stimulate your pineal gland—or open your "third eye," as it is referred to by mystics. The third eye is located in the center of your forehead, between your eyebrows. It symbolizes an opening of your inner vision to receive intuitive guidance from your higher power. Second, as I was later to discover, the humming technique massages the pituitary and thymus glands. The thymus gland monitors the production of T-cells and the pituitary gland monitors the elimination of toxins. Both glands are very important for the proper functioning of the immune system.

Sometime after my healing, I met two researchers who were

studying the effects of massage on the pituitary and thymus glands. When I told them about the humming section of the Nadabrahma, they suggested that the sound vibration performs an inner massage on those vital glands. I now teach this meditation to all who participate in my workshops and private sessions.

The Nadabrahma can be practiced alone or in a group. It is best performed on an empty stomach. It has four stages, and is designed to be practiced with specific music which supports each stage. The music also changes to indicate the transition from one stage to the other. (To purchase a Nadabrahma meditation tape, refer to the order form at the end of the book. The long version is one hour, the short version thirty minutes.) It is possible to do the Nadabrahma without the music on the audio tape. You will simply have to find another way to alert yourself when it is time to move on to the next stage.

FIRST STAGE: HUMMING. Sit in a relaxed position, with your spine erect and your eyes closed. When the music begins, inhale through your mouth and start to hum through your nose, with your lips together. The humming is like a monotone chant and should be loud enough that it creates a vibration throughout your entire body. Simply allow yourself to make a sound in your throat, but let it come when you exhale through your nose, creating a very nasal sound.

Visualize your body as a hollow tube or empty vessel through which the humming vibration flows. This vibration activates the brain, cleansing and rejuvenating each fiber. After a while you will reach a point when you become merely a witness, and the humming happens of its own accord.

You can alter the pitch and the pace of inhaling and humming, until you find a rhythm that is comfortable. If you need to shift your body to be more comfortable, do so slowly and gracefully, remaining in tune with the gentle flow of energy moving through you. Be sure to keep your spine erect, so that you can breathe fully.   30 minutes (short version 7½ minutes)

SECOND STAGE: GIVING. With your eyes still closed, stop humming and gently lift your hands so that they are at the level of your heart, with palms facing up. As the new music begins, very, very slowly allow your hands to move in an outward circular motion. The right hand moves to the right, and the left hand moves to the left. Make the circles large, and as slowly as possible. It is an allowing, not a doing. At times it may feel as if your hands are not moving at all, or that they are moving on their own. While your hands are moving, focus on giving your energy to the universe.   7½ minutes

THIRD STAGE: RECEIVING. When the music changes again, turn your hands palms down. Move your hands in the opposite direction, inwardly toward your body, in a circular motion. The right hand moves left and the left hand moves right. While allowing your hands to move as slowly as they can, focus on receiving energy from the universe.   7½ minutes

FOURTH STAGE: SILENCE. When the music stops, lie down on your back in an open position. Your eyes are closed and your body is perfectly still. Stay awake and alert during this stage. It is the most active stage of the meditation. It is the valley of expansion.   7½ minutes

19

The Healer Within

*Love is the most healing force in the world.
Nothing goes deeper than love; it heals not
only the body, not only the mind, but also
the soul. If one can love, then all one's
wounds disappear.*

—OSHO,
I Celebrate Myself

TO BE A HEALER really means not to do anything. The less you
use your mind and all its beliefs, the more healing is able to move
through you. God is the true healer. Healing is being whole with
God.

Within each and every one of us, there is a healer. It is the
intuitive part of us that guides us on our healing journey. It is an
intrinsic yet much forgotten aspect of ourselves. In fact, it has been
so neglected that it is considered highly mystical and esoteric by the
logical thinking of Western cultures.

We cannot connect with the healer via the mind, with its old
assumptions and expectations. The way of the healer is fresh and
new, coming from the mystery of each new moment. In fact, one of
the secrets of accessing the healer within is to let yourself be surprised.

The definition of a healing personality is the willingness to
take a risk, the risk to heal. It is the willingness to trust our intuitive
guidance even when we do not completely understand it. The healer
is the part of us that is willing to be inspired by life, with the
innocence and curiosity of the soul child. In order to return to that

natural state of grace, it is crucial that we empty ourselves of the old decisions and survival programs that clutter the way. We must be willing to go beyond logic.

I met my healer, or more precisely I stumbled onto my healer, several months after my diagnosis, because I could no longer endure the frustration of postponing living at my maximum potential. I knew that the time for indulgence was over. It was time to stop catering to the child survivor with all of her impossible needs and capricious whims. I was finished being run by her constant need to be "good" in order to belong. It gradually became more and more evident to me that the stressful energy of the child survivor was predominantly responsible for my physical body becoming susceptible to disease. The child survivor was also the part of me that was obstructing my journey back to health.

Giving My Child the Love She Craves

When I gave my inner child the unconditional love, genuine care, and nourishment she craved, she could begin to feel safe, and move out of survival mode. If I took care of her emotional needs myself, she would no longer need to "run the show" in search of the acceptance and the emotional strokes she felt she needed from others in order to survive.

In a painful way, I finally realized that the love she was looking for would have to come from within me. It was time to let myself love and provide for my inner child, so that she finally could let go of her hope that someday her savior would come, as all the fairy tales, love songs, and Hollywood movies had promised her. It was time to wake up to the real world, and to let go of the fantasies.

That is what the healer provides for us. It tears apart the dreams, the justifications, and the false hopes. It allows us to begin our healing journey by taking responsibility for our present situation and becoming creative.

Accepting Responsibility from Within

The healer is willing to accept life as it is, in the exhilaration of the unknown. The healer is willing to tell the truth, to ourselves and to those around us. It takes great courage to admit that we are an integral part of the cause of our present situation and that it didn't just happen to us as victims. The healer can see the ugliness of blame and the misuse of anger when it is directed at someone: anger then becomes useless and destructive. And it is the same with complaining: it only encourages the belief that we are helpless victims and that life is miserable.

In order to appreciate and be grateful for the simple and magnificent miracle of who we are and of the world around us, we must shed the mask of victim. The healer is willing to accept full responsibility for her life, embracing each event as another doorway to a deeper understanding of the inner self and the outer world.

For example, one of my clients decided to put himself in charge of whatever was happening to him. He made it clear to his doctors that, before anything was done to or with his body, he wanted to be informed precisely of all of the outside circumstances, concerns, and possible side-effects so that he could make all major decisions personally. He did not consider himself a passive patient, but a member of the team. In fact, he considered himself the captain, because, as he said, "The field that we were playing on is my body."

One of the keys to a healing personality is to have the courage to work as part of a team and to be willing to be in charge. This takes tremendous courage, because our "free" society is based on its members giving their power away to higher authority. It starts with the Judeo-Christian concept of God as an authority figure who punishes and forgives, and continues with our governmental leaders, our teachers, and our health practitioners.

Self-empowerment comes when we realize that healing energy originates from within and moves outward. Unfortunately, Western medicine approaches this upside-down. We are always looking outside ourselves for this pill or that method which will serve as the "magic bullet." I find this to be true even with alternative and metaphysical approaches.

Visualizations and Affirmations For example, when we practice visualizations and affirmations mechanically, by rote, because they are "good" for us, very little can happen. The mind is filled with subconscious programs which will sabotage the process. If you are affirming "I am healthy" over and over, yet you have a subconscious program that says "When I am sick I get attention," it will block the healing process.

On the other hand, when we are connected with the intuition of the healer, affirmations and visualizations come to us naturally, as if out of thin air, followed by a sense of empowerment to take action aligned with the understanding behind the affirmation. For example, "I am healthy" could translate into a natural desire to exercise and eat consciously.

Affirmations and visualizations are very powerful techniques to reeducate the mind, especially in connection to the body. Affirming a statement over and over as an acknowledgment of its truth affects our body, no matter whether it is a positive or negative statement. By using positive affirmations, we can release energy blocks created by old beliefs or decisions that are no longer appropriate today. Two positive affirmations that I use are: "I am now open to the healing energy of love" and "I now allow the Light to guide me on my path."

I recommend allowing affirmations to emerge naturally, in a relaxed way, as opposed to doing them in a mechanical manner. Each image is then created by your consciousness and fully received by your body. For example, my visualization of Niagara Falls was an image that my mind created spontaneously. Whenever you use affirmations or visualizations, it is very important to meditate first, and then visualize or repeat the affirmation, letting every image or word penetrate your mind and body. This requires total concentration, so it is best to practice this in a place where there is as little distraction as possible. If some disturbance does occur, include it in your experience. Do not resist it. If you hear barking dogs or police sirens, simply say yes to them as a part of your environment, and refocus on the positive affirmation.

I cannot emphasize how important it is to meditate and align your energy with your healer before using any healing technique, from positive affirmation to preventive medication. For instance, every time you take a pill, consciously empower it with the energy of your healer so that it can be more effective with fewer side-effects. Don't just pop it in your mouth unconsciously.

Proper Nutrition The same principle holds true for nutrition. Many of my clients follow strict macrobiotic diets, others follow proper food-combining guidelines. Some eat chicken and fish, while others drink wheatgrass juice. In a sense, it really doesn't matter. What matters most is that you discover what diet works for *you*. The beliefs and judgments you have about certain foods affect your digestive process in a positive or negative way. My guilt about eating chocolate, for example, was as stressful to my body as the sugar itself.

It is very empowering to be fully present in the moment when we are eating. It is important to prepare our food with love, beginning by choosing foods that we know will support our body, instead of indulging the inner child. When we sit down to partake in a meal, it is nice to bless the food with gratefulness, to thank Mother Earth from which it came. While eating, allow yourself to slow down and focus totally on the experience of eating. Take the time to taste the food. Chew the food well, one mouthful at a time, instead of rushing the experience as we have been conditioned to do in this fast-food society of ours.

To be fully present with your meal may mean not to watch television or read magazines (especially the news, or any AIDS-related information). When eating with others it may be helpful to eat in silence for part of the meal, so that each of you will be able to fully participate in eating and to align with the gentle rhythm of your digestive systems. What we put in our bodies is vitally important to our health, as are the attitudes we have about nutrition, and the awareness with which we practice it. Healing requires that you are awake and conscious of what you are doing every step of the way.

Connecting with the Healer

You may wonder how you are to know when you are connected with your inner healer. First of all, the healer lives in your heart, and exists only in the now. The healer offers words of wisdom in simple sentences without the need for long explanations. Her compassionate guidance creates a sense of expansion within you, and she is closely aligned with your soul child.

Here is a process to assist you in getting in touch with your healer. Trust yourself and your ability to communicate with her.

PROCESS

Connecting with the Healer Within

Let your eyes close, and take several deep breaths, letting yourself be exactly where you are right now. Don't try to change anything.

Continue to breathe deeply while you allow yourself to focus on the screen of your mind. Observe all the circumstances of your present life, no matter how challenging or overwhelming they may appear to your child. As you watch, simply let yourself be the witness, saying *yes* to whatever you are seeing. Then take another deep breath, and feel your *yes* even more. If a no comes, say *yes* to your no. Simply breathe and mentally say *yes*. If it comes naturally, let yourself whisper "Yes" aloud. Let your *Yes* grow, and fill all of your being. It is in your *yes* that you will meet your healer.

Let yourself be surprised by its form. It may be a particular color, such as violet, or a physical sensation, such as warmth, or even an archetypal or religious figure. Your healer will be unique to you. Once you have connected, let yourself and the healer spend time together. Explore your connection. Recognize each other. Dance together for as long as you wish.

When you feel totally connected with your healer, open your-self to receive an answer to a question that is important to you. Ask the question and silently listen to the gentle guidance of the healer within you.

Let yourself be surprised by the answer. Keep your energy high and alive. Stay light. When you feel complete, thank your healer for its love and guidance. Gently allow yourself to return to your body and to the present moment. Slowly let your eyes open, and write down the healer's guidance in your journal. Then take some quiet time alone to integrate the answers into your present life. It is then your responsibility to go for it, guided by your healer. Remember to reassure your child survivor that you are now in charge, and that you will take care of her, as you take this new direction together.

Some of you may have had a glimpse of a healer that did not fit your picture. When we begin to contact the healer, we often find not that big powerful savior who is going to magically make all of our problems go away. It's not the one who is going to desperately grab at all the solutions. It's not somebody who is going to take us by the hand and promise to show us the way to the end of the rainbow, where we will live happily ever after.

The healer within might appear as somebody extremely vul-nerable and honest. In the honesty of the moment, we may discover that we don't know who we are, and that that is the energy of the healer. The healer is something vulnerable and fragile which doesn't necessarily fit our child's expectations. In that vulnerability a different kind of strength is available, coming from acceptance instead of from defense. It is total honesty, without masks, pre-tense, or judgments.

If you were to ask the healer about whether or not to take a specific medication, for instance, the healer may answer, "I don't know, but I am willing to be here with you so that we can explore it together." The healer is open to what is so today, and what tomorrow will bring. She may not know what it is, but she is willing to be surprised.

We usually look for the healer to come from our old conditioning, from our mind, from the part of us that learned how to disconnect from the healer. Remember that the mind uses our assumptions and expectations to project our opinions from the past onto the present and future. We often miss the immediate recognition of the healer within, because it is a totally new energy. It is a simple beauty. When we are in touch with the healer, life becomes effortless. I am not suggesting that there are no obstacles or difficult moments, but there is rarely any resistance to them.

The Unconditional Compassion of the Healer

The energy of the healer is one of great compassion. Compassion is a doorway beyond judgments. I believe that compassion is one of the main qualities needed to heal ourselves and our planet. I was so quick to judge Nado as well as myself, despising the parts of us that needed healing. But the healer generates an experience of coming home to oneself by embracing all that we are and by accepting the parts that we were rejecting as well as the ones that we valued. In that embrace we find a really compassionate response in ourselves.

The wonderful aspect of the healer is that it is always available, and it is unconditional. My healer didn't tell me that I had to first heal my fear of the dark before she would be available to me; the healer is always there. The child survivor may push it aside because it doesn't fit her picture, but the healer remains faithfully. The healer waits patiently until that moment when we can begin to hear and trust its quiet voice above the chatter of all the other voices coming from the masks of the child survivor.

The Healer Versus the Child Survivor

The healer will always be available to you *except* at the level of the child survivor. This may be a frustrating statement, one that you don't want to hear. Of course, on one level, the child can serve a useful purpose, and often provides an opportunity for healing. You may have picked up this book, for example, because of her fear of death, yet the child survivor quickly becomes an obstacle to healing.

For example, when we have just received a diagnosis of a life-threatening illness, the fear of the child survivor motivates her to search for a solution that will avoid pain and death. The child survivor will do anything she can to fix the problem and make it go away. Because of this, she has a powerful instinct to find books, teachers, and methods that will help her avoid or postpone facing the fearful events of her past that stand in the way of healing.

The healer, on the other hand, is the one who directs us where to look, and shows us what action to take in order to reach our maximum potential. She guides us to take our next step no matter how uncomfortable it may be. The healer may suggest that we let go of our indulgence and completely change our way of living life. She may request that we clean up our act, our environment, and our relationship with the world.

The healer can also assist us in recognizing that we are the one resisting, we are the one complaining, and we are the one judging and abusing ourselves. It takes a lot of courage to finally let go of the "poor me" victim attitude, especially in our society. (Look at our judicial system, in which we can sue anyone for anything, and never assume responsibility for our actions.) The healer is willing to show us that the child survivor can be a master manipulator, always choosing to operate out of fear and refusing to accept responsibility for her life.

The moment in which we access the healer is often the beginning of an uncomfortable journey because it is a very new way of living life—transcending our old conditioning and our desire for control. The child survivor may feel cheated or deceived, or may resent the healer for asking him to change. This can also trigger anger, and that too is a part of healing. It gives us another opportunity to flush out anger.

In the beginning it may be difficult to recognize the difference between the child survivor, wearing the mask of the healer, and the healer itself. Meditation is the most effective tool to differentiate between these diametrically opposed energies. The healer is easily recognizable, because it feels like a "yes" energy which is very self-empowering. The child survivor feels like a "no" energy with all of her fear and resistance.

Often when we become acquainted with the very simple guidance of the healer, the child survivor may instantly rebuke it. For example, one of my clients was a heavy smoker. When she connected with her healer, her inner voice gently recommended that she stop smoking. The child survivor became annoyed, because she wanted to be able to continue smoking, even though she pretended that she was willing to do anything to heal. The child survivor was willing to run five miles every day, eat all natural foods, do yoga, meditate—anything besides giving up the harmful habit. This is another one of the strategies of the child survivor, who will endlessly bargain with you to avoid change—which she views as a survival threat—and to protect herself.

"Healing Stress"

I acknowledge the courage that it takes for anyone challenged by AIDS, ARC, or any other life-threatening illness to trust the guidance of their inner healer, when a barrage of other choices are constantly bombarding them. Many of my new clients arrive totally stressed out from navigating the ocean of decisions, or burned out because they tried to do everything, to be sure not to miss anything. Many are forced to choose between medications, both of which have severe side-effects.

It can be very scary to risk making the wrong decision when your life is on the line. I have noticed that people usually either follow to the letter what their doctor recommends, or choose the alternative path, exploring the myriad of choices available to them. These include anything from homeopathic herbs and remedies to experimental drugs and treatments. Many people faced with too many choices become overstressed by their fear of making the wrong decision. Others bounce from one treatment to another looking for the "magic cure."

When I am with clients who have reached this level of stress, I invite them to stop everything for a day or two. (Of course, certain medications cannot be discontinued casually, so I recommend that they check with their doctor first.) During the hiatus in their routine, I invite them to meditate frequently, so that they can reconnect with their healer within instead of being run by their terrified child. (If you find yourself suffering from "healing stress" you may want to try this process, but only with the mutual consent of your doctor and therapist. You can begin by using the above process to connect with your healer.)

Once they have reconnected with their healer, I recommend that they make a complete list of all the options presented to them. I invite them to tune in and see what resonates for them with a positive empowering energy, and what creates a sense of disempowerment and weakness in them. Then they can make their decision accordingly, knowing that decisions are not written in stone and fluctuate with the healing process.

If the choices are made in a context of integrity and self-empowerment, we gradually learn to trust the guidance of our healer unconditionally.

The healer is not concerned with making mistakes. She trusts that everything fits together in divine order. The healer is willing to stay in the question, and simply be guided by life itself. Trust is the key to the door of the healer. Trust and love are the main components of healing, and all the treatments and techniques we use are simply tools to return us to the wholeness where love resides.

PROCESS

Creating Your Own Prescription

As part of your healing journey, it is important that you create your own "prescription" for health. To do that, begin a dialogue with your healer, following the steps described above, and ask her for guidance. Then ask what ingredients will serve you in reaching your maximum potential, including tools such as meditation, diet, exercise, affirmations, and body work.

Write your prescription for health in your journal, including any words of guidance or support you may have received from your healer. Your "prescription" will be the foundation on which you will build your daily awareness routine.

20

Your Daily
Awareness Routine

Until one is committed,
there is hesitancy, the chance to draw back,
always ineffectiveness.
Concerning all acts of initiative (and creation)
there is one elementary truth,
the ignorance of which kills countless ideas
and splendid plans:
that the moment one definitely commits oneself,
then Providence moves too.
All sorts of things occur to help one
that would never have otherwise occurred . . .

W. H. MURRAY,
The Scottish Himalayan Expedition

I AM OFTEN ASKED what specific exercises I did to heal myself.
First of all, as I have said many times, I did not heal myself; it was
an allowing, not a doing. I allowed my body to heal itself by
listening to it carefully, and by no longer indulging my child survivor. Some of the specific ways I did that were:

- I learned to live in the moment.
- I reprioritized my life, putting myself on the top of the list.
- I learned how to be committed to myself, and created healthy
boundaries in my life.
- I slowed down my pace, and learned to say yes to the precious gift
of life, as it was offered to me moment by moment.
- I became a disciple of life, instead of of my neurosis.

■ I meditated daily for a minimum of one hour, sometimes for up to three hours.

■ I developed a dialogue with my inner child, and learned to embrace all of her.

■ I trusted my healer within.

■ I used visualizations and affirmations.

■ I exercised daily.

■ I changed both my physical and my mental diet, consciously choosing what I would eat, what I would read, and what I would watch at the movies or on TV.

■ I carefully chose whom I wanted to spend time with.

■ I created an honest and supportive relationship with my doctor, and trusted my intuition to abstain from any medication. (That was my personal choice, I don't necessarily advocate it for anyone else.)

■ I made sure everything around me, including the day-to-day details of life, measured up to my own personal standards.

Restructuring Your Life

Slowly the tools and techniques I had learned and taught at the ashram stopped being techniques and evolved into a way of living. My invitation to you is to begin to restructure your life to support your healing, by creating your own daily awareness routine using the guidelines of your prescription.

It is important to create this routine organically from your own flow of energy, and not mechanically impose it on yourself. Healing takes dedication, perseverance, and discipline. Many of us fall out of discipline fairly easily; therefore, creating a structure and sticking to it is very important. Sticking to the structure will train you to reprioritize your life and put yourself on the top of the list. Please respect the structure of your daily routine and follow it to the best of your ability. At the same time, be realistic about what you are creating, because even though it is good to stretch your limits, you must make sure it is reasonable. You do not want to set yourself up to fail.

It was not always easy to drag myself out of the warm comfort of my bed at dawn to meditate in front of the sunrise, but I knew the cost of listening to my voice of indulgence. I had made a commitment to myself to be bigger than that voice of indulgence, and to live from that commitment. On certain days it was not easy. Believe me, if I can do it, you can do it as well.

Following our own daily awareness routine is literally being willing to grow up and become an adult. By following a daily awareness routine, we become willing to be mature about our way of living, and embrace the principles that promote our maximum potential for health in our lives.

P R O C E S S

Creating Your Daily Awareness Routine

Tune in, and look at all the areas of your life, including your relationships, your job, your home, your finances, etc. . . . Open your journal and make a list of all of your daily activities, including work, play, personal hygiene, household chores, and spiritual discipline. Include what you enjoy as well as what you do begrudgingly.

When your list of daily activities is completed, prioritize it according to what is most important to you. Number each activity according to its importance, beginning with number one for the most important. Now open to the page on which you wrote your "prescription." See which tools you already practice, and which ingredients need to be added. Take the time to include the tools you want to integrate into your daily life, like meditation or exercise. This is the beginning of your daily awareness routine.

What a daily awareness routine provides is not necessarily a change of our circumstances, such as the child survivor would like, but a reprioritizing of our lives. Many of you do not have the ability to change drastically the circumstances of your life, and therefore it would not serve you to try. There may be some of you

who could use a change of environment, job, or relationship as
motivation to create a totally new lifestyle; if so, trust that. It
depends on what works for you. Remember to trust the guidance
of your inner healer regarding any changes.

Here is an example of what my daily awareness routine was:

6 A.M.	meditation
7:00	breakfast
7:30	take care of my body
9:00	set my three daily goals
9:15	do my household chores
11:15	rest
11:30	walk on the beach
12:15	rest
12:30	lunch
1 P.M.	continue daily chores, make phone calls, etc. . . .
3:00	meditation
3:30	work
5:00	meditation
6:00	dinner
7:00	open evening, friends visiting, reading, support groups, etc.
10:00	bedtime

PROCESS At the end of each day I would ask myself if I had
accomplished my three daily goals and complete with the question:
"What about today am I grateful for?"

Once you have designed your own daily awareness routine, make
a commitment to yourself to honor its presence in your life. This
commitment will assist you in remaining true to your healing journey, even when the child survivor would rather indulge or avoid.

My Commitment to Myself

I _____ make a commitment to myself to
do my daily awareness routine every day. I choose to go

beyond my limiting beliefs, and let go of my fears and conditions. I am willing to commit one hundred percent of my energy each day to each process and meditation I practice. I am willing to discover what it is to be grateful. I am willing to discover what it is to be new. I am willing to live in the question: "Will this action or attitude support my maximum potential?"

Keeping commitments nowadays is very rare. We are living in a society that has descended into indulgence. Divorce is commonplace. Killing is ordinary. Corruption does not even make us blink any longer. We have been so anesthetized by our environment that it takes great courage to be willing to stand up for ourselves and our integrity.

Another purpose of the daily awareness routine is to retrain ourselves to keep our word, not only with others, but with ourselves as well. For instance, I have worked with many clients who are completely reliable in their jobs and in their relationships with others, but are unable to keep commitments to themselves. This is another example of the child survivor running the show. She keeps her promises with others as a way to avoid rejection and gain approval. After years and years of doing for others while denying ourselves, we burn out and become resentful. If we keep our commitments to ourselves, then we will naturally and effortlessly keep our commitments with others.

I would like to share a quote by the great modern dance pioneer Martha Graham that inspires me to strive for my maximum potential. In 1945, Graham wrote, "I am a dancer. I believe that we learn by practice. Whether it means to learn to dance by practicing dancing or to live by practicing living, the principles are the same. In each, it is the performance or the dedicated, precise set of acts, physical or intellectual, from which comes shape of achievements, a sense of one being and a satisfaction of spirit. One becomes in some areas an athlete of God." In 1985 she reflected on her earlier words: "When I first wrote those lines some forty years ago, I little thought I would be looking back at what is now a sixty year history for my dance company. I still believe in that perfection which fights against what is for me the only sin, mediocrity."

Three Daily Goals

When we are sick, we need to rest, and our body needs to slow down, but often we confuse resting with inaction. By staying active, we stay interested.

As part of your daily awareness routine, I highly recommend that every day you choose three goals to accomplish. This process greatly assisted me in moving beyond my indulgence, and sometimes was the only reason I got out of bed in the morning. It will create a sense of personal victory in you and empower you to be in charge of your life. It will also help to strengthen the muscle of integrity within yourself and create a sense of expansion in your life.

For example, one of my clients had difficulty making it through the day without becoming discouraged and overwhelmed by the circumstances of his life. Between his doctor appointments, support groups, acupuncture, medication, and all the red tape required to receive his Social Security and insurance benefits, he had no energy left to do anything else. He began neglecting himself and his home.

When he first came to work with me, he perceived death as a welcome relief and just hoped that it would come quickly and painlessly. I could see that his desire for life was still present, but he was simply overwhelmed. He didn't know where to begin in order to accomplish what was ahead of him. I suggested that he make a list of all his tasks, including even the smallest details, like sewing a button on his jacket. When the list, which spanned several pages, was finished, he chose which tasks he wanted to accomplish that week, and divided them up into three goals per day. After only four days of keeping his word with himself by accomplishing his three daily goals, sometimes despite his resistance, he experienced a genuine joy and eagerness to accomplish more.

Working with Your Inner Child

The child survivor will tend to resist what is new, or what is "good for her," at first. Use the following sample checklist every week as a way of keeping yourself accountable with yourself. The checklist is also a useful tool to assist you in refining your daily awareness routine. At the end of each week you can readjust your schedule, dropping what you are willing to let go, and spending more time on the important tools.

Remember, as you do that, please be aware that the child survivor may try very hard to bring back some old indulgences into your new way of life. To avoid this tendency it is up to you to demonstrate to her, with great love and tenderness, that these changes are improving the quality of your life to support your healing. Share with her that this new way of living is the passage. If you gently guide her step by step into this newness, it will keep her interested. The inner child loves to learn, when you lovingly teach her without imposing any expectations on her. There have been enough expectations imposed on her already. Take the time to have a dialogue with her daily, during this period of transition. It will make your journey much more joyous and fluid.

This checklist is a supporting tool to witness your personal transformation. It is not an opportunity to make yourself wrong, and punish yourself. It is a useful tool to discover who you are, the illusions you have about yourself, and the emotional obstacles you are ready to overcome.

SAMPLE WEEKLY CHECKLIST

(Create your own to reflect your new life.)

In the table below, check off each task when you've completed it on a given day.

	M	T	W	TH	F	S	S
Daily meditation							
3 daily goals							
Did I live up to my maximum potential?							
Gratefulness process							
Inner child dialogue							

Tune in once a week to choose which goals you want to achieve in the different areas of your life for the coming week and write them in the Goal column below. Then include them in your 3 daily goals. As the week progresses, fill in the other two columns with your actions and the results they produce. Your daily goals may be the same every day, but the moment they become a routine, stretch yourself with new goals.

	GOAL	ACTION	RESULT
Physical body	_____	_____	_____
Relationship	_____	_____	_____
Work	_____	_____	_____
Home	_____	_____	_____
Recreation	_____	_____	_____
Spiritual	_____	_____	_____

I give myself a gold star for: _____

Being One-Hundred-Percent Committed

Nothing that is suggested in this book requires previous training, education, or experience. It only requires you and your total commitment and participation.

If you want to succeed in anything, it is very important to be one-hundred-percent committed and passionate about it. For example, look at the success of Madonna. She is so totally committed to everything she does. People believe that it is her singing or her dancing or her videos that are the keys to her success, but that is merely a superficial assessment. I believe that the real reason for her success is that she is passionate in every step she takes and every move she makes. It is true with all great artists. Look at Picasso, who was willing to go far beyond convention to express his truth. We recognize the greatness in artists like this, and they inspire us.

When you say yes to everything that life offers, it awakens a sense of passion and aliveness, and forces you to live in the now. If you are angry, be totally angry, let yourself disappear into it. If you are confused, let yourself be totally confused. If you love, let yourself melt totally in the love. If you hate, hate totally, not just a part of you but all of you. By saying yes we become passionate about life and death.

It is in our passion that the healer within us emerges, the child survivor disappears, and compassion becomes present. Being passionate is a key to healing. Most of us resist what life offers us. We want it to be different, but then we miss. For example, we may wake up in the middle of the night, feeling fear and anxiety, and we resist it. It doesn't fit our self-imposed schedule. We take a sleeping pill in order to control what life is offering us. We judge it as bad, and we miss what would have happened as a result of our insomnia. Perhaps it would have been a great awareness, the answer to our prayers creeping quietly into our mind in the middle of the night.

Being passionate and saying yes to life means going with the flow. It takes great courage to do that. Being one-hundred-percent committed will attract a lot of judgment from the people around us, because their way of partial commitment and half-truths is so much safer. The healing path is a courageous journey, and once you have embarked on it there is no turning back.

As you do your daily awareness routine, you will open up to dimensions of understanding that go beyond the old logic that you are used to living with. It is important that you trust this evolutionary process and be willing to move in those new directions as they organically evolve.

Keep It to Yourself

I invite you to keep your daily awareness routine private, especially in the beginning. This is for the simple reason that most of the time when we share something new and often quite inexplicable, we open ourselves to the skepticism or the negativity of others. Until your new tools, habits, and understandings are fully integrated into your daily routine, there is no need to expose your fragile newness to unnecessary "putdowns." So please keep your healing journey to yourself unless you are asked by someone who is open and willing to receive what you have to share.

Your Healing Community

One place to share your journey is in workshops and support groups. I cannot emphasize enough how important it is in the beginning to participate in a healing community, which is gently guided by an appropriate facilitator for your journey. At first you may not want to participate actively, and that is fine. Just by being there, you will have a taste of the supportive energy. It is nearly impossible to create that supportive energy by yourself, especially if you don't yet know what it feels like. If you are challenged by AIDS, cancer, Epstein-Barr, or any other life-threatening illness, find a support group that will provide a network of doctors, therapists, nutritionists, acupuncturists, and body workers who specialize in working with people facing the same challenge.

Healing circles and support groups are a beautiful place to begin, but as you grow the longing to fully blossom may surface. Then it is your responsibility to find the right community and environment where conscious, gracious living is present. These places are rare, yet very needed, and that's why I created the Healing Home.

21

Pain and Obstacles

Mountains fall and seas divide
before the one who in his stride
takes the hard road day by day,
sweeping obstacles away.
Believe in yourself and in your plan,
say not, I cannot but I can,
the prizes of life we fail to win,
because we doubt the power within.

—ANONYMOUS

MANY OF YOU challenged by AIDS might be just beginning your healing journey, and it will take tremendous courage to continue. I invite you to let every opportunistic infection be another opportunity to go deeper into the discovery of yourself.

For some of you, the middle of the journey, when the enthusiasm of the newness fades, may be extremely challenging. It takes a great commitment to continue living with integrity in spite of the child survivor, who may tell you to give up.

One of the first discoveries on the healing journey is that even when we "do the right thing," such as trusting our inner healer, and respecting our bodies, our pain does not disappear overnight. No matter how hard we try to be positive, obstacles such as an opportunistic infection still show up in our lives. We also discover that, even when we are challenged by a disease, our bills still keep coming, our relationships still have their ups and downs, and we still may not be getting the simple love and care we long for.

The child survivor will use this rationale to return to the old, comfortable way of living. For example, I have observed many clients who have flashes of great insight and self-discovery, but whose understandings melt away like April snow when an opportunistic disease invades their body. "Oh my God," I've heard people say, "that work didn't mean anything. All that meditation is hoo-ha. It doesn't really work." This is the reaction of the child survivor, who is attached to specific results.

The moment the child survivor doesn't get what she wants, she either complains, blames, or manipulates. This only creates more pain and obstacles, and makes us a victim. Then there is no room for the healing which comes from the mastery of acceptance. When we say yes, letting the creativity of our healer guide us, and allowing ourselves to make mistakes, we become masters of our lives. Pain is transformed into emotion and obstacles become challenges.

The Magic Bullet

One of the biggest obstacles to healing is the search for the "magic bullet," and the challenge is to realize that it does not exist. Many people have come to work with me because of the disappearance of HIV in my system, hoping to find the trick to accomplish what I did. Of course it is the child survivor desperately searching for the miracle cure, who leads these people to me, and frankly, within the context of our conditioning, this is a healthy response. In medical schools across the country our future doctors are learning that there are two ways of healing: chemical or surgical. That's it. That's the choice. Nowhere is there any acknowledgment of the healing power within us.

I was lecturing one evening to a group of people with AIDS about my healing journey, and a very intense young woman interrupted me. "Niro," she said, "all of this is beautiful, but right now I am waiting for the results to my HIV antibody test and if

I have that thing in my system, I want to get rid of it. I want the magic bullet." I said, "Okay, imagine that I have given it to you and AIDS is now a thing of the past, then what?" She blushed, and told us, "If it were really out of my system I would quit smoking, move out of New York City, try to be closer with my family, and dedicate my life to help others, oh yeah, and finally grow the roses I have always wanted to grow." "You just described your magic bullet," I said.

Right away she responded with, "Yes but . . ." I invited her to stop for a moment, drop the "but," and really receive what she had just shared. We all watched her silently for a moment. She slowly began to weep as she understood the misleading road she was on and her fear of starting to live the vision in her heart for herself and the world.

It is very difficult finally to let go of our reasons for postponing the discovery of who we are, and then actually to live in the light of that discovery. When we finally surrender fully to the truth that "I probably will die from this disease—and if not I definitely will die from something, when my time comes," then we can begin to live our life fully, from conscious choice, instead of in our unconscious state of sleepwalking.

The New Age Trap

Another obstacle on the healing journey is what I call the New Age trap. This is a misinterpretation of higher truths by our child survivor. For example, in New Age philosophy we are repeatedly taught that we create "our own reality," which logically would include our disease. Yet this truth in the hands of the child survivor results in her punishing herself or grabbing a new hope of doing it "right."

I've heard clients say, "If I created this disease, then I should be able to heal myself of it." Of course on a soul level we create everything in our life and healing involves taking responsibility for this. Yet if the child survivor is allowed to misuse that higher truth, it only creates guilt and "healing stress."

For example, I have encountered many people who feel like failures because they were unable to love their disease like so many New Age "healers" invite them to do. They ask me, "Niro, how did you learn to love your disease?" I tell them that I never loved it. In fact I still don't love it. The truth is I hate it, but I recognize it as one of the most powerful teachers in my life. I never tried to change my reaction, yet transformation still took place. That is the mystery of the journey.

The New Age Pusher Often, in response to healing stress, the child survivor will don the mask of what I call the New Age pusher. She will do anything to avoid pain and death, including pretending to be spiritual. She may use New Age tools in order to "accept" something she really hates. She'll do endless meditations, visualizations, and affirmations, and usually ends up feeling lost, doubting herself, and resenting the tools. She literally tries to learn how to lie to herself in order to do what she thinks she "should" do to be spiritual, moving farther and farther from her own truth.

My invitation to you is this—don't try to accept circumstances you hate. Accept how you feel in connection with your circumstances. Accept your anger. Accept your hate. Don't pretend it's not there. Simply observing what is so is the beginning of the spiritual journey. Learning to love yourself exactly as you are is the first step to enlightenment.

The Trap of Forgiveness I see the same trap with forgiveness. Many people do exercises on forgiveness, repeating "I forgive myself" over and over like a mantra. Yet often when they are in my workshop they realize they are still carrying a lot of resentment toward a specific person or issue. The forgiveness exercise might have created a sense of expansion in the beginning, but it usually does not last.

It also does not really promote healing, because it is not their truth. Their truth (or more accurately their child's truth) is often angry, resentful, and even hateful. Doing those exercises when the child's feelings have not been acknowledged first is just a way of covering it up. It is the mask of the controller, doing the right thing in order to protect herself. Remember, forgiveness is not a "doing." It is the fruit of being in harmony with ourselves. Forgiveness has many levels. It may take time to reach that stage of self-acceptance and let go of the past. Only then can true forgiveness really blossom. Be patient.

The Mask of Bliss In the New Age trap I constantly see people wearing the mask of expansion and bliss, hoping that mimicking it will help them attain it. It is another survival tool of the child trying to belong and avoid rejection. The consequence of this trap is being fooled by our own mask into thinking that we have reached some destination, and that this is where our journey of discovering ends. Healing takes a willingness to remain humble, open, and vulnerable, staying in the question instead of settling for easy answers. This can be very difficult because of our attachments to our relationships, our ambitions, our achievements, and our material possessions.

On our healing journey, it is important to be aware of our attachments to comfort, to the old. Whenever we begin to feel too comfortable, it's time to wake up and snap out of it because most of the time comfort is a sign that we have fallen asleep again. Our child survivor will often find a way to escape the discomfort of staying open and vulnerable by wearing the mask of the healer. She will justify our actions by explaining how important it is for us to avoid whatever feels uncomfortable. For example, one client's child survivor was a master at playing the role of his "higher self," who would persuade him not to attend our support groups. Later, in a private session, we discovered that his advice was actually coming from the mask of the child survivor. It was his way of protecting himself, because he was uncomfortable with the unfamiliar experience of unconditional love that was available in the support group. The child survivor will use any excuse, and wear any mask including that of the healer, if it will help him to do his job of protecting us from harm, or to be more precise, trying to make us invulnerable.

Whenever we find ourselves in this New Age trap—and most of us have been there at one point or another—we need to recognize that we are wearing a mask, let it drop, and rediscover our vulnerability. It is through the fragile opening of the heart that we can experience the real nectar of forgiveness, peace, and freedom.

"Cashing In" on Disease

Another trap that the child survivor may fall into is using disease as manipulation to get his needs met. For example, he may use it as an excuse not to work, or as a way to be taken care of by his partner or by society. Basically it is another device to avoid accepting personal responsibility. This can be dangerous, because if we are receiving "goodies" in return for being sick, it will empower the disease within us.

For instance, I have observed that many people with AIDS who participate in the self-healing workshops I facilitate request scholarships. Of course some of them literally are physically unable to work, and are living on minimum Social Security or disability pensions. This, combined with exorbitant medical and pharmaceutical bills, creates a real need for financial assistance, which we provide for them. There are others, however, who are HIV-positive but asymptomatic. They request scholarships because they are unemployed, or "broke." This feeds the child survivor who will use his illness to get things for free, manipulate those around him, and try to get what he longs for. There is a clever part of every one of us that enjoys a certain sense of power when we get something for free, but is totally oblivious to the real price we are paying for it.

We might be able to cheat Uncle Sam for a few thousand, but then we wonder why our car is mysteriously vandalized in a parking lot, or why we lost our wallet. Karmically, it is all connected as in a gigantic jigsaw puzzle. We never get something for free. Only the mind feeds that belief. Because the strategies of the child survivor are not very mature, the superficial expansion that "getting by" creates can lead to very dangerous habits. This behavior is a covert way to celebrate disease, and it respects the victim more than it does the creator in our lives. If we receive too much without having to earn it, then our creative energy dissolves from misuse and the motivation to reach our maximum potential disappears very fast.

I see an interesting correlation between opportunistic disease and the opportunist in us who survives by "cashing in" on being sick. I remember one very young client who had recently been diagnosed HIV-positive but was asymptomatic. He took a paid leave of absence, which was covered by his insurance, in order to integrate the news and reconcile his life. Within three weeks, he had applied for and received a fifty-percent discount subway pass because of his "disability." When he told me, I felt an immense sadness, but I refrained from saying anything.

During our session, I invited him to engage in dialogue with his child survivor. He discovered that his child was so afraid of the uncertainty of the future that every penny he could save created a sense of security. Because his child was so fearful, his controller asked him to cut out all luxuries like travel or entertainment. The controller nearly requested that he stop eating and using the phone—anything that would create bills. When he switched back to the present adult, he was very surprised by the reaction of his child. He realized that his child survivor was preparing for disease without even questioning the reality of it in his present life. By getting his discount pass, he was already perceiving himself as a sick person. By denying the joy of being alive and full of energy, by not celebrating his ability to pay the full fare, he was making the disease more real.

The Obstacle of Separation

Another obstacle we encounter when faced with a life-threatening illness is the feeling that we have become different and separate. We often feel it right at the moment when we receive our diagnosis, our wake-up call. There is now a difference between us and the rest of the population, who have not received a life-threatening diagnosis.

This is partly due to the fact that we now have different priorities than the majority of people. When we recognize that we are now different, it is important not to consider ourselves "wrong." This leads to the tendency to isolate ourselves in our misery.

Isolation is not the same as aloneness, which is a conscious choice to take the inner journey of self-discovery, a journey that can only be made alone. Isolation is often a reaction to the fear of rejection. One area in which this can be particularly painful for people with AIDS is in terms of sex and relationships.

Sex, Relationships, and HIV

Dealing with sex relationships and intimacy is another frightening obstacle we encounter following an HIV diagnosis. It is usually based on the fear that sex and relationships will no longer be part of our lives.

It is very scary the first time we have to announce our health status to our sex partner; our libido can be adversely affected by the newness of the situation. All we can see is what we've lost and that our old ways of relating are now gone. Many people prefer to stop dating for a while. Some return to it later in safer climates such as support groups and other HIV-positive meetings designed to facilitate that process. For example, PWA coalitions across the country organize tea dances and other social events specifically for HIV-positive people.

Heterosexual Women Heterosexual women who are given an HIV-positive diagnosis seem to react very differently than gay men do.

I see many of them withdraw and "make themselves wrong." Most of the HIV-positive women I have met fell easily into the belief that relationships were now something of the past. This is partly due to the fact that most HIV-negative heterosexual men will not generate a relationship with someone who is HIV-positive.

Yet isolation and celibacy does not have to be the only solution for HIV-positive heterosexual women. I have seen many exquisite relationships blossom out of the connections made in my workshops. This is partly because my workshops are a very safe place, where we can be open to the truth of what is happening right in the moment. When people meet in the moment, in a safe environment, their health status is not at the forefront of their interactions. It does not invalidate the depth of their connection. For instance, a man and woman who are both HIV-positive met in my support group and are now happily married.

Creative Sex We need to become creative as we learn to practice safe sex, and this takes time. Changing our sexual habits can be disturbing, especially in long-term relationships. For example, one of my female clients, who had been infected by a blood transfusion, suffered tremendous shame because her husband was unable to have intercourse with her any longer.

When this happened it was very difficult for her to trust that she was still loved, since the demonstration of affection she was accustomed to had changed. Through working together in a support group, she and her husband began a healthy dialogue with each other. They learned how to express their true feelings, including their sense of helplessness and their fear of AIDS, instead of pretending that these feelings were not there, and avoiding each other. Today they have a creative partnership in discovering who they are in relationship to each other and in their ever-changing life circumstances. This has created a shared intimacy that is much deeper than it ever was in their entire married life together.

It is very helpful, when you or your partner is faced with an HIV-positive diagnosis, to create a climate where intimacy can develop in other shared activities of your lives—enjoying quality time together, dining, dancing, taking evening strolls, hugging, massaging, or any number of creative options.

There are also several creative safe sex options available, including the discovery of mutual masturbation. With the gentle guidance of your love for each other, you will slowly find new ways of connecting. The art of tantra is a magnificent door to a new dimension between two people. Riding the wave of sexual energy through the technique of deep breathing increases your energy instead of decreasing it. Together you will be mutually nourished far more than is possible through ordinary sexual intercourse.

Because of society's repression of the subject of sex, most of us grew up feeling insecure or self-conscious on some level about our own sexuality. Therefore when you are challenged by a sexually transmitted disease such as AIDS or herpes, it is important to stay as present as possible with your feelings. Allow yourself to witness your emotions and say yes to the fear. This will assist you in moving through the potential misery of your child survivor. Many of my clients who had the courage to say yes to their feelings have transcended their fear and are now in more intimate, more sexually alive relationships than before their diagnosis.

Turning Obstacles into Challenges

If we begin to consider obstacles as challenges that we may resist at first, but that we inevitably will accept, we can begin to shift our perception, opening ourselves to learn from them. Just look back at events in your life that at the time seemed unsurvivable, but which somehow you survived. Here you are reading these words, perhaps carrying a scar, but still very much alive.

It is my belief that, when it is time for us to move on to the next life, there is very little we can do to change it. We may think that we can control our circumstances, but as we have seen, that is an idea of the victim, not of the healer. The healer knows we have no control over certain passages in our life, and that we must simply surrender.

What we can change is our attitude, which directly affects the way we respond to obstacles. The difference between an obstacle and a challenge is very subtle, and we must stay awake in order to recognize it. The way to detect this difference is so simple that we might not trust it at the beginning. When we perceive an event as an obstacle, we usually avoid it, but when faced by a challenge we are interested. An obstacle creates a "no" energy and a challenge creates the energy of "yes."

When we perceive a challenge as an obstacle, we resist it. The more we resist it, the more real we make it. When we resist pain, we make it seem worse, as often happens when we visit the dentist. When we can say yes to the pain, this allows the pain to move. By letting go and relaxing, we let the pain dissipate more quickly.

Physical Pain

It does not matter whether the pain or disease is physical or emotional, the obstacles are still the same. Probably the most confrontational obstacle of all is the fear of suffering from physical pain. Many of us are more afraid of physical pain than of death itself. This is an area where it is important to acknowledge our limitations and recognize that the extreme approach rarely works. When we are willing to keep meeting the pain moment by moment, we can determine the appropriate use of medication. It is a process of awareness through acceptance.

The fear of pain is sometimes more paralyzing than physical pain itself. The process of connecting with our pain, learning our limits, and meeting the "coward" in us is also a part of the bumpy road to enlightenment that our body is taking us on. Often we learn to be in the now like never before. When we are affected by physical pain, our entire awareness is focused on it. We often forget about all of the other past and future circumstances of our lives. We have an extended experience of being present because there is no way not to be when we are in pain (if we don't suppress the pain with painkillers). Often without realizing it, we have surrendered to the moment while we wait for the pain to subside.

Medical science has been extremely helpful in the area of physical pain, yet sometimes this is dangerous as well, because we learn to rely on it so quickly. When we immediately suppress the physical pain, we risk missing the lesson that it is there to teach us. Some people try to abstain completely from painkiller, with a nearly martyrlike attitude, while others go to the opposite extreme, requesting morphine at the first sign of physical pain. I'm not advocating one way or the other—the use of painkiller is a very personal choice—but extremes rarely work.

The best way to deal with physical pain is to let ourselves experience it fully and completely. This facilitates the movement of its energy. Unfortunately, this often goes directly against our instinct to hold our breath and tense our body, to keep the pain at a distance. (Remember, when I had those strange attacks of throbbing pain all over my body, I would stop everything, close my eyes, and breathe deeply. This would allow the pain to be released.)

At the beginning the pain may feel like a concrete block of dark energy. But when we are willing to stay with it, simply breathing into it, we may be surprised that this solid mass may become less dense. It might move from dark to less dark. It may even pulsate in rhythm with our heart or our breath. As we focus on this pulsation, we become aware that the pain is moving, and the body will respond to this flux immediately if we simply allow the physical experience of contraction and expansion to develop. The more we can go with it, the more the pain can move. This is where the mystery lies. A sense of relief may come very rapidly, and we can nearly fall into a restful state. Or the pain may grow more intense for a while, finally reaching a peak, before it will swing into a valley, allowing the body to rest.

PROCESS

Embracing Physical Pain

Please ask someone you feel very comfortable with to lead you in this process. Choose someone you trust, for this journey is a very private one. There is no right or wrong way to do this process, except to put yourself into it as completely as you can and remain true to yourself. There is no need to perform for anyone. If it is easier, you can record the process yourself, and then listen to it as you play it back in your own voice.

Lie down on your back on your bed and close your eyes.

The following text should be read aloud by a friend:

"Please breathe deeply and bring your full attention to your breath. Let yourself feel your own presence to the best of your ability. Become aware of what is happening in and around you. The sounds, the smells, the sensations."

(Pause.)

"Now open up and go beyond your five senses. Let yourself be open to your intuition and to guidance from your inner healer. As you continue to breathe deeply, begin to focus on the light within. Visualize a beautiful, shimmering white light, representing the presence of God. Trust whatever image your subconscious brings forth; this is simply a guideline. The color may be purple or blue or green, just let it be whatever it is. Let yourself be in the presence of God. Let the light bathe you."

(Pause.)

"As you begin to feel safe and your body becomes more and more relaxed, become aware of the center of the pain that is affecting you."

(Take a deep breath.)

"As you continue to breathe, let the light enter your body and comfort you. Let the comforting sensation fill all the parts of your body that are *not* in pain, so that the painful area becomes more and more precise. Bring your full awareness to the center of your pain. Feel the specific location of the pain and notice how it feels different from the rest of your body."

(Pause.)

"Now allow yourself to draw healing energy and strength from the parts of your body that are not in pain. Request God's guidance and support in this process."

(Take a deep breath.)

"Continue to breathe deeply as you go deeper and deeper into the pain. It might be very scary, as if the pain will be too much. Trust the guidance of God, and keep on going. Now you can only feel the pain in its full intensity.

"Remember to continue to breathe deeply even though your tendency will be to tense up and hold your breath. Now observe what color the pain is. Trust whatever image comes."

(Pause.)

"Now what is the dimension of it?"

(Pause.)

"What is its form?"

(Pause.)

"What is its size?"

"As you continue to breathe, see the pain in its full reality. Keep focusing on the form, size, and intensity of the pain. Your body may want to cry, let it cry, or scream or sigh. Simply let it happen. Let the energy move.

"Now, asking for the full assistance of the light within you, and using your full creative power, see the pain become smaller, the color paler, and the intensity softer."

(Take a deep breath).

"Feel the pain now. Maybe it is throbbing. If it is, feel the pulse. Watch its dance of contraction and expansion. The intensity followed by stillness, in and out, in and out. Feel the pain beginning to be supple. Again with the guidance of God, and at your own pace, use your creative power to visualize the pain becoming smaller."

(Take a deep breath).

"As the pain diminishes, let yourself rest in the lesser intensity of the pain. Simply concentrate on your breath and on your body resting on your bed. Give yourself a break. Let your body take a break."

(Pause.)

"Now once again, using your creative power, visualize the light inside of you, healing the pain completely, and let yourself fall into a state of rest. Let yourself be with God. God is always ready, always there for us. We need only to get out of the way. It is our choice to remember that we can let go. We do not have to suffer. We can be open to the support of our friends and loved ones, as well as to God. Let yourself spend time in deep appreciation of yourself and of God."

PROCESS

Dialogue with Your Virus (or Condition)

(Read the entire process first before you do it.)

Prepare yourself for a dialogue with your child as usual, but this time put two cushions or chairs in front of you.

Begin by centering yourself as the present adult, bringing your full awareness to the position of your body, your presence in the room, and rhythm of your breath.

It is very empowering to start this particular process with a short dialogue with your inner child. Simply explain to her what you are about to do, including her in the process. If she is frightened, it is your role to reassure her. Make it clear to her that you will not abandon her.

Following the dialogue with your child, return to the present adult. Now focus on the second cushion or chair in front of you. Visualize your virus or condition in front of you, as an individual entity that will speak to you using your voice.

A powerful way to start this dialogue is to directly ask: "What are you doing in my body?" or "in my life?" Remember that it is important to center yourself first and ask the question as invitingly as possible.

Remember that you are about to meet something that is confusing to the child. She sees it as a friend who gets her attention, as well as an enemy which brings suffering and consequences that she has no notion of how to handle.

Let the virus or condition be as articulate as possible. If it is answering something that the present adult does not understand fully, switch, and ask for clarification out loud, then switch back. Keep the dialogue alive by taking regular deep breaths in order to stay in an expansive, receiving state. If you feel resistance or contraction, check in with your child and see if she needs to express herself.

Here's an example of how the dialogue might go.

PRESENT ADULT: Hi, virus, I would like to ask you some very important questions. The first one is, why are you in my body?
[*Physically switch and become that entity in your body.*]

VIRUS: I am here to teach you love.

[*Switch.*]

P.A.: I don't understand. I have done a lot of work on myself, and I was under the impression that love is what has been guiding me how to live. Can you explain what you mean?

[*Switch.*]

V: Yes, it is true, but you have never included yourself in the way you live, and it is not healthy. It is time for you to learn self-love.

[*I feel resistance to the answer, so I switch to my child survivor, who wants to ask a question.*]

P.A.: Can my child ask you a question?

[*Switch.*]

V: Yes.

[*Switch again.*]

CHILD SURVIVOR: What do you mean? You are making me very uncomfortable. I feel I don't really know what you are talking about and that makes me afraid.

[*The child may need to express how much she does not want the virus there, and how frightened she is of the virus. Let yourself express anything that you have been keeping inside for so long.*]

[*Switch.*]

V: We are taking a journey together. I came into your life because somehow you were not conscious of your purpose here. I did not come to harm you. I am sorry your body is going through an uncomfortable passage. Please understand that you really need to begin to live in a totally different way, in a way that is much closer to your soul. You need to begin to love and respect yourself. Otherwise you are living in a split, in a separation between yourself and your soul. This is the source of my presence. Please begin exploring the love you have for yourself.

[*The information resonates in me and I know it is the truth, so I return to my present adult.*]

P.A.: I will, even though I'm not yet sure I know how.

Allow the dialogue to end naturally on its own. Remember to finish in the present adult mode and to take the time to be grateful to yourself, your child, and the virus for being so open. Spend some time feeling gratitude for the deep transformation that has taken place. At the end of the process, rest in the emptiness of having expressed your questions and received your answers.

This process can be done regularly, as part of your daily awareness routine.

22

Death: A Completion
of Life

*My tongue is getting numb and I cannot
say anything more, but remember, up to
now I am as whole as I have ever been.
Nothing has died in me. Something has
died around me, on the periphery, but in
contrast the center is in fact more alive
than ever. I feel more alive because the
body is dead, all the life has become con-
centrated. It has disappeared from the
body, from the circumference. It has become focused on a single point: I am.*

—SOCRATES' LAST WORDS

UP TILL NOW I've told you about my personal experience of
healing. Now we have come to a topic with which I have no personal experience, except as a witness—death. As I shared earlier,
death doesn't frighten me as much as the fear of suffering does. I
feel ready to welcome death with open arms when it comes. Since
it is my goal to be fully present in the moment of death, I want to
ride that last wave of life as a magnificent surfer, using my fear of
the unknown and my love of life to support the passage.

Through the ages many enlightened masters have taught that
meditation and death are very similar experiences. In death, the
ego-personality (child survivor) disappears, and only pure being
remains. The same happens in deep meditation. In India, it is called

samadhi. In Japan it is called satori. It is like my experience on the beach. The separate personality melts into pure is-ness. The "I" disappears, and like a raindrop returning to the ocean, it merges with the whole. This is what the masters have said death is like. It is the dropping of the container of the body and the cup of the mind, allowing the river of our essence to return to the ocean of God. Death is like meditation. This is why meditation prepares us for death.

I have so many friends on the "other side" that it has taught me the importance of expressing my feelings to my dear ones while they are still alive: We never know when it will be too late. I try not to have any unfinished business with anyone. My diagnosis taught me the value of living with the fragile awareness of the shadow of death.

I do not see death as the end, but as the culmination of life. It is the climax. Of course, when a loved one dies I grieve the passing, but I have discovered that I can choose to stay miserable or to embrace the presence of that person's energy in my life. So many of my friends and clients have been important teachers to me, revealing new understandings about the mystery of death. They are still vividly with me every time I speak on the subject of death in workshops and lectures, and I would like to share some of their inspiring passages from this life to the next. (I have changed their names to protect everyone's privacy.)

Darkness into Light

When I started working with David, he was surrounded with a dark feeling and was terrified of death. He could not even say the word without getting near hysterical. Driven by his terror, he began his healing journey with a very deep commitment. He meditated regularly, and practiced his daily awareness routine religiously. In a few months his life was totally changed.

He had always wanted to return to Europe, yet postponed the trip numerous times due to financial considerations and other excuses. One day in session he realized that returning to Europe symbolized an important step to him. It was more than just a vacation. He decided to give himself this experience and traveled throughout Europe for several months.

While he was there, he visited the tomb of Napoleon and had a transcendental experience. He understood that death was merely a passage and that what really mattered was how one lives. He also woke up to the fact that he had been unconsciously choosing to live in fear, and from that moment on he chose to live in love. That love had always been inside of him, but he had hid it all of his life.

Now, David's light shone brightly and his love overflowed, touching everyone around him until the day he died. On that day, shortly before his passage, his relatives asked him how he was doing. He was unable to speak, but he looked up at them and smiled, making the okay sign with his fingers.

Going Home

Another of my clients, who became a very dear friend, was also terrified by death when I first met him. Chris was afraid of dying young and of the pain it would cause his mother.

Chris was a very sensitive man and a spiritual seeker most of his life. His healing journey was very intense, but regardless of how many opportunistic diseases he was challenged with he kept bouncing back from one after the other. Toward the end of his life he was battling CMV (cytomegalovirus) and was confronted with the possibility of losing his physical sight.

One day Chris shared with me his fear of going blind and his new appreciation of his sight, which he had taken for granted for so many years. He was really looking at flowers like never before. He also shared that if he were to lose his vision he would learn to touch the flowers and discover them from a totally new perspective. When I heard that, I was inspired and moved with a sense of deep respect.

When I first began working with Chris, he was in love with

someone who would not commit himself, and he longed to be in a real relationship. It was very painful for him, but with each session he was able gradually to accept that his friend Tom was not ready.

Several months later they did my workshop together. After one of the processes, Tom realized that it was his child's fear of commitment that was preventing him from opening up and letting Chris into his heart. Tom then courageously chose to surrender to his true feelings, and they entered into a committed relationship. They were so beautiful together. There was so much love and understanding between them.

According to Tom, on the last morning of Chris's life, Tom asked Chris if he should stay home or go to work. Chris responded that he should go to work as usual. When Tom was ready to depart for work, he asked Chris, who was resting in bed, how he looked. Chris responded with a loving smile and softly said, "You look beautiful."

Shortly thereafter, while Tom was at work, Chris told his caregiver that he wanted to go home. The caregiver reassured him that he was home. Chris shook his head and said, "No, I am going Home." He then gently closed his eyes and stopped breathing.

Letting Go into Death

One of the participants in my first ten-week course was someone very inspiring. His death taught me the level of a person's commitment toward the people who love him.

As a child, Wayne had made a subconscious decision that it was very important to behave well. He was one of the most considerate and reliable persons you could ever meet. He was in a relationship for twelve years with someone very beautiful, whom I'll call Greg. They both had been living with AIDS for four years. Toward the end of Wayne's life, it seemed that the road they had shared for so long was coming to a fork. It was time for them to go different directions.

During one of my workshops, Wayne discovered a part of

himself that he had buried at a very early age, who spoke his native tongue. In a dialogue process he was able to meet the mother who had abandoned him, and forgive her as part of his completion. Later he shared with me that he was willing to accept the different direction that Greg was taking. It was very clear to me that he was complete with relationships in general and had no interest in another one.

It had always been very important to the controller in him that he do things "right." But as part of his completion process, preparing him for the passage from life to death, he subconsciously let himself completely go. He let his body lose control of everything, including his bowel movements. Because of Wayne's fear of abandonment, Greg lovingly reassured him that no matter what happened he would not abandon him. His surrender was complete, and an inspiration to those who witnessed it. During the last three days, Wayne consciously existed in the zone between life and death, explaining to Greg what he was seeing, sometimes in his native language and sometimes in some other unintelligible language that only he understood. His friends were with him round the clock until the morning of the third day. By "coincidence" it was very early in the morning and he was alone with his lover. Wayne regained consciousness for a few moments, smiled at Greg, and gently left his body. He had completed with this world and inspired many of us through his healing into life and death.

Dying in Resistance

One of my most difficult lessons was with one of my closest friends. I had to learn to let go and allow her to make her own choices, and still be true to myself when in her presence. Our relationship became very tense, but was always honest. Because it seemed to me that she was making all the wrong choices, I judged her as a kamikaze who was consciously choosing to sabotage her journey, using very destructive tools.

Every time I went to see her, I found it an enormous challenge to accept her choices, and not try to "rescue" her. She literally chain-smoked, setting her bed on fire several times, after having quit for many months. The moment she started smoking again, she changed from being very light and accepting to destroying herself through constant justification of her addiction.

She was able to persuade her doctor to give her morphine, which she abused even when she was not in pain, because she feared the pain. I am still angry at her doctor for allowing her to become an addict again after fourteen years of sobriety. She had been an inspiring and vibrant woman who would often share her incredible recovery from drug addiction with others who were recovering. Now I had to watch her return to her own private hell.

I did whatever I could to refrain from judging her, but continued to remind her that there were other options available. I shared with her that I was still able to see who she was, and respected whatever her choices were. Deep in my soul, however, I could not agree with them. Her resistance to death taught me so much. For one thing, I learned how to move beyond my righteous judgment of what is "right" or "wrong" and just accept her as she was. I learned to put my "doer" and my "fixer" on the side, and always maintain my heart connection with her. I learned about the helplessness of both the caregiver and the care receiver. I also became a witness to how much drugs contaminate a person and everything around them.

Several months earlier, before her relapse into drugs, she had shared how much she wanted to be fully present at the moment of death, with her dear friends around her. Instead she chose to die alone. The last time I saw her she grabbed my wrists and held them so tightly that my blood was unable to circulate. She was fighting, resisting death all the way. When her kidneys failed, her doctors were amazed that she lived as long as she did. She fought until the very end, unable to trust that the passage would be beautiful.

I still feel a deep sorrow and a sense of failure about her passing. Yet I am grateful to her, because her death forces me to live at another level where I can accept the unacceptable and embrace it as a part of the cosmic puzzle of the universe.

Suicide: The Ultimate Form of Control

Many of my clients faced with painful and debilitating symptoms, and with very little hope for recuperation, have asked my opinion on suicide, and I am usually reluctant to answer. Suicide is the ultimate way of controlling life. It is the final tool of the child survivor to escape fear and pain. If we choose to kill ourselves now, then we don't have to face the unknown.

Personally I believe that suicide should be the last possible method of dealing with the pain of disease and dying. This is because the presence of each of us on this planet is a collective as well as an individual experiment. Part of this experiment we call life on earth is to make peace with the transition of death. This is extremely difficult since the global consciousness feeds our fear of death, which begins as a basic survival instinct and then becomes a lifelong obsession for many of us. For some, the fear is so intense that they would rather control the time and circumstance of their death than allow it to happen in its natural course.

I have discovered along my healing journey that life never sends us a challenge we cannot handle. It is very easy to disagree with that point of view unless you have survived a major crisis. For instance, if the survivors of the concentration camps during World War II had been asked if they would be able to live through the horrors they were about to face, they most likely would have responded with a definite no. But our inner resources become available in a crisis situation.

Yet who am I to judge another person's decision to end his or her life? I don't believe that suicide is a moral question that should be decided by governmental or religious law, I believe it is ultimately a personal decision. It requires tremendous compassion on the part of those who are left behind to accept such a choice.

"No Point in Saying No to My Destiny"

Another dear friend and client experienced an illuminating healing in the midst of his suicide attempts. Doug was a very exquisite being who was emaciated and close to death when he first came to work with me. During the ten-week course, he was admitted to the hospital with an opportunistic infection and we all thought he would die. It had been his goal to be fully aware of "receiving" his death, in a state of peaceful completion. While in the hospital, he became aware that his desire to die was actually an escape from what his life had become. He decided that he didn't want to die that way, and three months later he was a changed man.

Doug lived the remainder of his life to his maximum potential. He gained weight and exercised, redeveloping his beautiful physique. He would arrive for sessions with me on roller skates, vibrant and alive, overflowing with light. His positive effect on those around him was inspirational.

Yet, as so often happens to people with AIDS, six months later he was back in the hospital with another opportunistic infection. While there, he would travel from room to room, dragging his I.V. bottle with him and sharing his love and light with the other patients. Eventually he lived as an outpatient, receiving periodic chemotherapy treatments and completing with his family and friends. He also spent a lot of time in solitude, completing with himself.

Those of us who loved him knew the end was near. One night, while celebrating his last birthday, Doug looked around at all of us before blowing out the candles on his cake. It was his way of consciously bidding farewell to each of us, and we all got it. Soon after, he departed for a retreat on a small tropical island. He wanted to live out the remainder of his life in a warm, beautiful environment.

One evening he called me from his island paradise to inform me, "Tonight is the night." I asked him what he meant and he told me he was going for a swim and that he would not be returning. I thanked him for sharing it with me, and told him that I respected whatever decision he made in his life. I asked him to make sure he felt complete in all areas of his life, though, before he carried out his decision.

Inside of me, I felt a strong sense of compassion mixed with doubt and confusion. I asked my higher power for inner guidance and remembered what Osho used to say. "Compassion is not having a bleeding heart full of sympathy for others, but it is a depth of love that makes one willing to do whatever is necessary to bring awareness to a situation." Suddenly I heard myself telling Doug, "If at any point the ocean becomes your enemy, I think it would be wise to come back to shore." After saying good-bye, I spent the night crying and meditating on the beach under a full moon.

The following morning I phoned to see whether by any chance Doug would answer, and he did. He laughed as he shared that, the more water he swallowed, the stronger he felt. In the middle of it he realized how ridiculous the whole idea was. He swam back to shore with the little energy he still had left, and wrapped himself in a blanket.

Several days later he swallowed enough sleeping pills to kill a horse, but that suicide attempt did not work either. Finally, he shared with me: "There is nowhere to go. No way out. No point in saying no to my destiny."

He decided to let nature take its course and surrendered to the idea of dying fully present in the moment when his time came. Nine days later he died in bliss. His road to a peaceful death had been quite bumpy and often very painful, yet through it all he never denied what was happening to his body, or his imminent death. He admitted that it had been his terrified inner child who had tried to end his life prematurely. The last time I spoke with him by phone, I told him how much it inspired me to be a witness to his living and dying fully present in the moment. He was no longer able to speak, but responded with a sound filled with so much love and joy that I interpreted as a jubilant "Yes!"

Death: A Door to the Divine

Osho once shared his feelings on death upon hearing the news of the death of a loved one: "Whenever somebody dies, somebody you have known, loved and lived with, somebody who has become part of your being, something in you also dies. Of course you will miss her, a vacuum will be felt, it's natural. But the same vacuum can be converted into a door. And death is a door to God. Death is the only phenomenon left which is not corrupted by man. Otherwise man has corrupted everything, polluted everything. Only death still remains virgin, uncorrupted, untouched by the hands of man. Man remains at a loss as to what to do with death. He cannot understand it, he cannot make a science out of it; that's why death is still uncorrupted, and that is the only thing left pure now in the world."

The concept of death can be totally liberating when we feel complete with life, even if there is still a part of us that would like to stay here in the garden of earth and play with our friends. Nevertheless, once we have put our life in order and completed the business we came here to accomplish, death is no longer the enemy. It is simply the next step in this adventure called life.

If we feel that there is still unfinished business, it is important to take the time to complete with the people, places, and things in our lives. The less baggage we are attached to at the time of our passage, the higher we can fly.

PROCESS

A Completion

This process is for everybody regardless of whether you believe the end of your life is near, for we all are going to die someday. Close your eyes for a moment and tune in to the areas of your life that still need completing.

The following questions will assist you in looking over your life, and in a simple way, discovering what needs to be done for you to feel complete. For example, it is never too late to tell someone how much you appreciate the contribution they have made in your life. It is never too late to tell someone that you let go and forgive. It is never too late to open your heart and live from love, compassion, and respect toward yourself and others.

Give yourself the opportunity to respond to each of the following questions in your journal. This is a very private journey, so again, do this process somewhere where you will not be disturbed. After completing this questionnaire, simply see which action you still need to take in order to feel complete. This will not only make your passage, whenever it comes, a more peaceful one, but it will embellish the days that remain with more love and compassion.

1. How fully have I lived my life?
2. Now that I know I will die, what are my current priorities? (Remember we are all going to die eventually.)
3. Who and what have been my teachers?
4. What still remains unfinished in my life with regards to:
   (a) my relationships?
   (b) my work?
   (c) my aloneness?
5. Who have I not yet forgiven? What must I do to complete with them?
6. How do I feel about myself at this moment of my life?
7. Taking an overview of my life, what was my purpose in being here?
8. In completing my life, what am I grateful for?
9. Looking back at my life, I acknowledge myself for . . .

My Understanding
of AIDS

Rather than a soul in a body,
become a body in a soul.
Reach for your soul.
Reach even farther.

—GARY ZUKAV,
The Seat of the Soul

WHEN I FIRST became aware of AIDS, it was something that was happening to other people, very far away from me. Of course there was no way to avoid the terrible atmosphere of panic and doom created by the media and reinforced by the masses, since it permeated the very air we breathed. Yet my attitude was the common one of avoidance, since it was happening to "them" and not me.

Even though I considered myself "spiritually evolved" and believed I was dedicated to making a difference in the world, I was just as much a coward as anyone else. I was afraid to open my eyes to the impact of such an epidemic on the world at large, and I did not want to face my personal fears and judgments about disease and dying. Little did I know that AIDS was to become my greatest teacher.

On a larger scale, AIDS has detonated a bomb under the surface of society with all of its collective fears and judgments. I have not met anyone who has remained indifferent to AIDS. Some may be judgmental, terrified, or even self-righteous about it, while others may be open, compassionate, and sincerely supportive. Either way, everyone has a reaction to it. AIDS has created a healing momentum on our planet. Virtually every level of our society is affected by it. It is the beginning of the drastic change that needs to happen on our planet.

Our planet, Mother Earth, is suffering from AIDS herself. Her breath (our air), her blood (our water), and her flesh (our land) have been polluted by little parasites called human beings. The immune system of our planet has severely deteriorated through years of abuse, neglect, and exploitation. The time bomb is ticking, and it is literally our wake-up call.

I believe that AIDS is the most powerful transformational tool that has ever been available to us on a mass level. It is forcing us to reevaluate the entire foundation of life as we know it. It is shaking the medical community and its related industries, it is affecting the educational and judicial systems. It is forcing us to question our values, our morals, and our identities. It is challenging us to treat our fellow human beings with compassion and understanding. This is the message of AIDS.

The tragically slow and incompetent manner in which our political and medical establishments have responded to the AIDS crisis is a clear indication of how sick we are as a collective culture. Darwin's survival of the fittest, in the urban jungles of our day, was never more evident than in the way in which people reacted to this human crisis. We were all a part of the fear and panic, sparked by the media's irresponsible and dangerously sensational handling of the story. We are all responsible for the heinous discrimination against people suffering with this debilitating disease.

Even though at the time we knew very little about the transmission of AIDS, the lack of compassion and consideration by the caregivers who refused to bring food into patients' rooms, of the ambulance drivers who refused to transport patients, and of the family members who refused to visit their dying loved ones contributed on some level to the emotional suffering and premature death of many people with AIDS. These are all symptoms of a sick society.

While watching Nado wither away and die, I swore I would

do whatever I could to help shift people's attitude about AIDS from one of panic and hopelessness to one of openness, to viewing this crisis as an opportunity for healing for anyone touched by it. I'm sure there are many other people affected by their loved ones' suffering and death from AIDS who made the same vow. In fact, it was these very people, working mainly as volunteers, who become the backbone of vital support services for PWAs. I would like to extend my personal admiration and respect to all those people who were courageous enough to transcend the early hysteria and provide quality loving service to their patients, families, and friends.

I am pleased to report that, as of this writing, the tide has turned and AIDS is no longer considered one-hundred-percent fatal. It is now classified as a chronic condition, with hundreds of long-term survivors living full, valuable, and inspirational lives.

My understanding of AIDS on a global level is that it is a doorway to facilitate the evolution of humanity on this planet. A great healing is taking place globally, even if it appears to be happening only individually. As each of us heals, we are helping to heal the planet. Much like an ant that performs its separate task as part of the greater whole, we each participate in the evolution of humanity in our own unique way.

As Gary Zukav explained in his book *The Seat of the Soul*, we are evolving from a species that seeks external power based on the five senses into a species that embraces authentic power based on a multisensorial awareness. This new awareness is more closely aligned with the energy of the soul. One way is not better than the other. The new way is simply the next step in the evolution of humankind.

I can absolutely say, from my personal experience, that self-healing is a direct result of shifting into this multisensory approach to living. This new approach includes our five senses but is not limited to them. It expands to embrace intuition, and our connection with God, or a Higher Power, or the Divine, whatever name you give it.

As of this writing, I have worked with hundreds of people with AIDS. These wonderful people, and many others like them, are at the forefront of this shift in human consciousness. They are all part of the reshaping of our collective unconscious, returning us closer to the energy of our Soul.

In speaking with them, I have discovered a very high level of integrity in each one, no matter whether they are from a privileged level of our society or are junkies in a ghetto. Whenever I ask them why they are here in this life, their response is invariably the same: "I am here to serve." As an example of this dedication to service, I cite all of the long-term survivors I have met and worked with.

Each one of them dedicates a large portion of their time and energy volunteering for AIDS organizations, or facilitating support groups, or speaking out against the government policy and the FDA's connection with the pharmaceutical industry, or just being there as a supportive friend and a good listener. I would like to emphasize that each of them attributes their willingness to serve others as a major ingredient of their long-term survival. They also acknowledge their fighting spirit, their creative partnership with their doctors, and their own version of a daily awareness routine (good nutrition, exercise, meditation, visualization, low stress, a positive attitude, and acceptance of their journey). Invariably these people have taken the leap beyond logic, beyond their physical challenge, and are living life to the fullest. In doing so they are transforming the world around them in a very powerful way.

I have the privilege of witnessing transformation on a daily basis as part of my work, when my clients accept their condition as an opportunity to wake up and live from the higher wisdom of their souls. As their hearts open, their love overflows and touches the people around them, opening their own hearts as well, and on and on and on . . .

Hopefully you can see that we are transforming ourselves, and our planet. Life has sent us a powerful wake-up call, and sometimes we wish it could be different. But God works in mysterious ways, and we grow in mysterious ways as well.

So let your heart open and be inspired by who you are—by who *we* are—and then see what happens. Are you willing? Do you dare say yes to the whole experience?

Go for it.

Suggested Reading List

Badgley, Laurence, M.D. *Healing AIDS Naturally.* Human Energy Press: Suite D, 370 West San Bruno Avenue, San Bruno, California 94066. 1987.

Beattie, Melody. *Codependent No More.* Center City, Minnesota: Hazelden. 1987.

Cohen, Alan, M.A. *Setting the Seen: Creative Visualization for Healing.* Eden Publishing Company: South Kortright, New York 13842. 1982.

* Cousins, Norman. *Anatomy of an Illness.* New York: Bantam Books. 1983.

Davar, Bob Owen. *Roger's Recovery from AIDS.* P.O. Box 6310, Malibu, California 90265.

Ferguson, Marilyn. *The Aquarian Conspiracy.* Los Angeles: J. P. Tarcher, Inc. 1987.

Fritz, Robert. *The Path of Least Resistance.* DMA, Inc.: 9 Pickering Way, Salem, Massachusetts 01970. 1989.

Gawain, Shakti. *Creative Visualization.* Whatever Publishing, Inc.: P.O. Box 137, Mill Valley, California 94942.

Harrison, John, M.D. *Love Your Disease.* Santa Monica: Hay House, Inc. 1988.

Hay, Louise L. *You Can Heal Your Life.* Coleman Publishing: 99 Milbar Boulevard, Farmingdale, New York 11735. 1987.

* Recommended that these titles are read first.

King, Serge. *Imagineering for Health*. Wheaton, IL: Theos Publishing House, 1981.

Levine, Stephen. *A Gradual Awakening*. New York: Doubleday/ Anchor Press. 1989.

———. *Who Dies?* New York: Doubleday/Anchor Press, 1989.

Matthews-Simonton, Stephanie. *The Healing Family*. New York: Bantam Books. 1989.

Melton, George R. with Wil Garcia. *Beyond AIDS, A Journey into Healing*. Brotherhood Press: 279 South Beverly Drive, Suite 185, Beverly Hills, California 90212. 1988.

* Rajneesh, Bhagwan Shree. *The Book of Wisdom*, Volume 1. Rajneesh Foundation International: 1983.

———. *Death, The Greatest Fiction*. Cologne: The Rebel Publishing House.

Russell, Peter. *The Global Brain*. Los Angeles: J. P. Tarcher, Inc. 1983.

* Schaef, Ann Wilson. *Escape from Intimacy*. New York: Harper & Row. 1989.

———. *Women's Reality*. New York: Harper & Row. 1986.

Shealy, C. Norman, M.D., Ph.D., and Caroline M. Myss, M.A. *AIDS: Passageway to Transformation*. Stillpoint Publishing: Box 640 Meetinghouse Road, Walpole, New Hampshire 03608. 1984.

Siegel, Bernie S., M.D. *Love, Medicine, and Miracles*. New York: Harper & Row, 1988.

Simonton, O. Carl, M.D., Stephanie Matthews-Simonton, and Creighton, James L. *Getting Well Again*. New York: Bantam Books. 1982.

* Zukav, Gary. *The Seat of the Soul*. New York: Simon & Schuster/ Fireside. 1989.

For further information
regarding tapes, lectures, and workshops
write to:

Niro Asistent
Box 255
East Hampton, NY 11937